# Signs and Wonders

# Signs
# and
# Wonders

UNDERSTANDING
THE LANGUAGE OF GOD

ALBERT CLAYTON GAULDEN

**ATRIA** BOOKS

New York  London  Toronto  Sydney  Singapore

*Author's Note:*

Please note that throughout the text, I've used the male pronoun He
to refer to God, but choose whatever fits your understanding of God.

ATRIA BOOKS

1230 Avenue of the Americas
New York, NY 10020

Library of Congress Control Number: 2002104346

ISBN: 0-7434-4642-9

First Atria Books hardcover printing January 2003

10  9  8  7  6  5  4  3  2  1

**ATRIA** BOOKS is a trademark of Simon & Schuster, Inc.

For information regarding special discounts for bulk purchases,
please contact Simon & Schuster Special Sales at 1-800-456-6798
or business@simonandschuster.com

Printed in the U.S.A.

*To Leonora Hornblow, Joann Davis, and Scott Carney*

# Contents

PART II:
BREAKING THROUGH TO THE NEW LANGUAGE

PART III:
IMPROVING YOUR RECEPTION
OF THE NEW LANGUAGE

PART IV:
THE POWER AND PROMISE
OF THE NEW LANGUAGE

PART V:
QUESTIONS AND ANSWERS
ABOUT THE NEW LANGUAGE

PART VI:
RESOURCES

# Foreword

THE CASE STUDIES and examples in this book are based on real people and events. The stories presented herein have been altered to disguise the identities of the people involved. Some are presented as composites and reflect the experience of more than one individual.

# Introduction

MANY YEARS AGO, after a long series of personal struggles and horrendous heartache, I began to experience God's presence in my life and my life improved dramatically. I believe God wants us to have our own personal tie to Him, to benefit from His direct guidance and love. For the last sixteen years, as founder and director of the Sedona Intensive, I have dedicated myself to helping people achieve this goal. Now, in this book, I offer my thoughts and ideas to you.

The centerpiece of my recent work is a concept I call the new language. The new language is God's mother tongue, the way God speaks to us in a nonverbal way through coincidences, synchronicities, angel murmurs, thought impressions, telepathy, signs and wonders, and other manifestations. God has been speaking to us in this symbolic language since the time of Abraham and Moses, but in the march of progress and the rise of science, technology, and institutional religion, we have lost our sense of the profound mystery of divine intervention.

In the work I do with clients who come to see me in the spectacular Red Rocks, I have been trying to resurrect the new language. My hunch is that the new language is the way we can deal with the dissonance we feel as we seek true spirituality. While mainstream religion most assuredly has its place, among my clients I find a surge of longing to reclaim personal power and remove the intermediaries who have stood between God and us as gatekeepers of our spirituality. My motto is "Let the power pass from the few to the many." The key to having direct access to God is improving our communication skills. If prayer is about talking to God, the new language is a divine answering system.

The new language is by no means all I teach in Sedona in my one-on-one personal-growth program. I focus on helping individuals clear away the static of negative emotions and difficult childhoods that keep us from hearing God's voice. I hope to take you by the hand and walk you though a process of clearing that I use in my work with the exercises, anecdotes, and practical instruction I provide in these pages. Clearing helps to heighten our reception of the new language by releasing us from the past, and centering us in the present, with increased awareness.

In this book, which is more than an exercise and instruction manual, I have tried to offer what has worked for me and hundreds of men and women whose lives have been transformed at the Sedona Intensive. James Redfield, a graduate of the Sedona Intensive, stimulated the imagination of millions of readers worldwide in his bestseller, The Celestine Prophecy, which he wrote after his trip to Sedona. How was he moved to write such a book? I will share this and more with you.

As you strive to break free of the limits you've set for yourself, and embrace what God has in mind for your life, remember that He is all around you with road signs of encouragement when you lose your way. What is most reassuring to me is that there are no calendars and clocks for enlightenment. The lightbulb goes on when you are ready to see what God is trying to show you and to hear His voice in the new language.

" . . . and he worketh signs and wonders in heaven and in earth . . ."
—Daniel 6:27


"I and the children whom the Lord hath given me are for signs and wonders."
—Isaiah 8:18


"Let the power pass from the few to the many."
—Albert Clayton Gaulden

PART I

*Listening for the Voice*

CHAPTER I

# What Do You See? What Do You Hear? What Do You Feel?

WHEN SUSAN RECEIVED WORD that she had been admitted to both Harvard University and Brown University, she asked her father for help in making the choice. "Both schools are excellent," he said, "but I think you should sleep on the decision." No sooner had he said the words than the doorbell rang. At the door was a deliveryman who said he was lost and needed directions. He was wearing a sweatshirt that carried one word in large crimson type: Harvard.

David was restless. Things weren't going well for him at work and with a big client meeting the next day, he was finding it difficult to sleep. Staring at the ceiling at 4 A.M., he was overcome by a powerful urge to turn on the radio. Following his intuition, he clicked a button and heard Bob Marley's voice chanting over and over again, "Everything is gonna be all right, everything is gonna be all right." Calmed by the rhythm, he fell back to sleep.

Barreling along in pouring rain, Michael was lost on an unfamiliar road. He had just been to the doctor's office to get his test results and the news was not good. "Please, God, help me," he was pleading over and over in his head. "If there's anything else I can do, please show me the way." The screeching siren that pierced his thoughts came from a police car pulling Michael over to the side of the road. Despite the light beaming out from the officer's flashlight, Michael was still able to see the billboard in the background, which read, Miracles Can Happen. Do Not Despair.

Are these coincidences? Signs? Messages? In my opinion, all of the above. I believe God was speaking to Susan, to David, and to Michael in the new language; that is, God's mother tongue, the way He's been talking to us since Biblical times.

Going as far back as Moses and the burning bush, God has been using sign language to get through to us. In the Bible story that is told in Exodus, Moses was tending his flock in the desert when he came to the mountain of Horeb. Now, in my opinion, Moses must have been a very clever fellow, because when God showed him a burning bush in the middle of the desert, he didn't miss a beat— Moses knew that God was speaking and wanted him to help set the Israelites free.

When Noah, his family, and the animals marched off the ark after forty days and forty nights of rain, God sent a rainbow as a covenant between Him and the souls who would replenish the earth. Noah understood. Later on, Abraham saw a ram as he was about to sacrifice his son Isaac and knew God had other plans.

After Biblical times, organized religions began springing up around the world. I believe this may be when the direct connection between God and mankind was interrupted. As early religions took root, the power became concentrated in a few hands. A hierarchy was established, with priests, rabbis, seers, and others acting as middlemen between God and us. The power brokers and other self-anointed intermediaries clearly enjoyed telling the rest of the folks what to think and what to do. A great many man-made rules and dogmas were established, and in no time people were down on their knees reciting the "right" prayers at the "right" time of day— as if God were an obsessive-compulsive ego who kept a tight schedule. The God who had made man in His divine image must have had a real chuckle as He watched man remaking Him along human lines. Did God stop talking because man wasn't listening? It's hard to know, but there seems to have been a suppression of the language. Church and state were virtually the same for thousands of years, and people in fear for their lives became parrots to the position of whatever government or religious institution was in power.

As time moved on, the Western world was plunged into the Dark Ages. During this 1,000-year stretch, none save Joan of Arc reported getting any news from God—and she came to an unenviable fate. While Joan was being tied to the stake and torched, most people were off fighting holy wars that meant death and havoc for millions of others.

When the Enlightenment arrived in the seventeenth century, the rational mind was emphasized, giving way to the rise of science. There is no denying that science has brought tremendous advances to health care and the workplace—we owe so much to conveniences and technology. However, most scientists are absolutely useless when it comes to the spiritual needs of society, perhaps because they can't test, measure, or dissect them. Truth for them has to be weighed and tabulated. Launching the technological revolution, the scientists put machines first. They substituted the rhythm of the machine for the rhythm of the soul. Anyone who has seen the great Charlie Chaplin movie *Modern Times* will know what I mean. A man on the assembly line becomes a slave to the clock.

After the assembly line, the conveyor belt, and the atom bomb came the revival in the 1970s of nineteenth-century Prussian philosopher Frederich Nietzsche's declamation that "God is dead," which may have unwittingly triggered the fighting spirit in the rest of us to discover our true spirituality. Our soul was crying out to recover.

And, in fact, we are recovering. The shift is now occurring. Since the middle of the twentieth century, when the human-potential movement began, we have been searching to find our way back to God. Fueled by a deep and unsatisfied craving, an awareness that the power must pass from the few to the many has been growing. Many of us want to control our own spiritual destiny, even if we enjoy participating in spiritual community and worship. On a very intuitive level, we want to have our own conversation with God, a more direct tie as Moses had. Spurred on by Freud and Jung, who deepened our self-knowledge, we have figured out that if we tame the ego we can become our very best selves, our spiritual selves, and be in an ongoing dialogue with the wonderful God who is there to help and guide us.

With His incredible sense of timing, God knows that the shift is taking place and He is aware of the window of opportunity that opened with the dawn of the new millennium. Ever ready to welcome us back, God has a whole repertory of techniques He is using to get our attention. He uses so-called coincidences and synchronicities—unplanned interactions between two or more people—and His messages are carried to us at very important moments in books and billboards, in poems and on the radio. God finds us where we live and He is definitely multimedia. Some may say this is all wild and crazy wishful thinking, the product of my vivid imagination. But I will tell you that to dismiss what I'm saying is to miss out on an extraordinary relationship with God that can bring you guidance, strength, and peace of mind.

## Pain and Suffering

Humans are the souls who choose to come to earth to learn and grow by taking on a physical body. Earth is a school with stiff requirements for the souls who make the trip. First of all, every soul has a lesson plan, and pain and suffering are the teachers. Nobody on earth escapes heartache. Pain seems to be the hallmark of the human condition. But if you stop and think about it, pain can be a blessing in disguise. Pain tests our attitudes. It often sneaks up on us and strikes when we least expect it. Will we be models of optimism like Michael J. Fox, who called his autobiography about living with Parkinson's disease *Lucky Man*? Or will we allow adversity to crush us? We have a choice.

Pain provides us with an opportunity to discover our strengths, to help us stretch and grow, to realize that we are spiritual beings with great powers. If we are anything like one of my favorite characters, Dorothy in *The Wizard of Oz*, the pain helps us to realize there's no place like home. Through suffering, we reach out for help and try to get back to the source.

## Divine Energy

Mrs. Schuler, who taught Sunday School when I was a boy growing up in Baptist Birmingham, had some very fixed views about God. She conveyed an impression of God as an old man with a long, white beard sitting in a big gold throne holding the Judgment book in His hand. Those who see God this way have my respect, but my vision has changed dramatically in my six decades of life. I now see God as a vortex of energy—pure, powerful, and the source of all life, including our own. Being of God makes each of us an indestructible bit of divine energy—a soul, if you will.

In the earth school, where pain is the teacher, energy is the unifying force. Energy is not only the basis of all solid matter—it's also the substance out of which all of our emotions and thoughts are made. That's why it is so important to be mindful of what we think and feel, to be constructive with our thoughts and emotions, and not let grievances and ill intentions hang over us.

The tiny, energetic pulses radiating out of our hearts and our minds can carry a positive or a negative charge. That charge influences both the force field around us as well as the larger universe.

Einstein said we live in an energy universe, and, of course, we do. Matter is energy slowed down, and massive energy is released when the smallest particles of matter are divided. Each human being is a divinely charged energy system, part of God's cosmic design. When you share what is in your heart with someone else, there is an energy exchange as emotions pass between two people. When you make love, that, too, is an energy exchange, an intermingling of force fields. Energy is also involved in some of life's darker transactions. When one person manipulates another person, that is an energy grab. Perhaps you've met an energy vampire—someone you feel sucks you dry each time you meet or talk. Energy is really at the bottom of a great many activities because that is God's design and we are His work of art.

The new language, God's language, is also an energy system—a divine one—that can be useful in encouraging us, making us feel connected, and steering us in the right direction. Our task is to engage the energy flow. As we begin our journey of discovery of how to do this, here is one secret word that I offer to anyone in need of help: Ask. Remember that line in the Bible, "Ask and you shall receive"? Well, when you aren't sure if you are headed in the right direction, ask for help. Ask often and with an open heart. Throughout each day, check in with God and see what you hear or see or learn. Become sensitive to the new language and the guidance it offers. Like any skill, your sensitivity to God's guidance will develop slowly and with practice. That's the journey we are going on in this book. Clearing, listening, practicing, and refining our skills.

Now, in the interest of full disclosure, I have a confession to make. I didn't always know this language and how to use it to hear

God—to go where He led, to do what He told me was wise. It took a long time for me to get there. And I still make a lot of mistakes. I was the prodigal child and I went astray. I had a lot to learn. A wise man once said that we teach what we need to learn. So, let's begin with my story, how I came to clear and eventually hear God in the language I speak today.

# CHAPTER 2

# Blanche and the Angels

BLANCHE IRONED FOR MY FAMILY every Wednesday. Poor people in the forties couldn't afford automobiles, so she rode the streetcar from the ghetto to our apartment in Elyton Village, a federally funded public-housing development in Birmingham, Alabama, known as the Projects. Back then, my family used public transportation for the same reason Blanche did—we were poor and had no alternative.

Living in Elyton Village was tough on me, a sensitive child easily upset by gruff talk and rough play. The brick-and-asphalt jungle full of families trying to cope with life after the Depression spooked me. Because I had been born with clubfeet, I was not an athletic child, so the community center that beckoned my brothers and sisters to sporting events held no appeal for me. I much preferred staying at home, especially when Blanche was there, washing and ironing and baring her soul.

"Child, I am mighty grateful to your momma for this job," she once said with a smile that expressed the appreciation she felt for the chance to come to our house and spend time with me. "You are a fine young man."

Growing up, I remember summertimes with Blanche vividly. Each Wednesday, from mid-June when school let out until classes resumed in early September, I would peer out of Momma's bedroom window and watch Blanche walking toward our building in her print housedress, always carrying a shopping bag and an umbrella—rain or shine. Her gray hair was tied in a bun crowning a face that conveyed a no-nonsense attitude laced with dignity. She always walked tall.

"Mr. Albert?" she would call when she came in the door.

Having seen her coming, I was on my way to greet her, ready for our familiar ritual. To begin, Blanche ironed and sang spirituals while I read my books. Then, after I had put away the clothes, clutching each warm piece as if it were part of her, I would hope for a little time to talk before she departed. I'd plant my elbows at the end of the ironing board and confide what was going on in my life—mostly the problems that stemmed from feeling lonely.

"What's wrong with me?" I would ask. "I'm not like the other kids. I don't feel like I belong." Blanche listened and then held forth.

"There's nothing wrong with you, sweet thing. You are like that litter of pups I had last week. Four of them were brown as your momma's head, and one was spotted. He was different, and that's the one I love the most. Don't ask me why, but it is the truth."

Years later, after I had struggled with a sense of right and wrong clouded by alcoholism, I would hear Blanche's voice and cling to the life raft of words that came to me in her many sermons.

"There isn't anything in this world that God can't fix. But He's busy. Real busy. So He has angels that come around and talk in your head. They make things all right, Mr. Albert. They make things all right."

"How do you know when it's His angels trying to talk to you, Blanche?"

"You know when you get the tingle. From your head to your toes you tingle. The angels take you over."

Blanche died in the seventies. I was living in California at the time and could not return home for her funeral. I had made several bad turns in my life and gone down some very mean roads. But her words still rang in my head.

# CHAPTER 3

# When Things Fall Apart

I WILL NEVER FORGET my first taste of alcohol.

It was 1957. I had dropped out of college in an attempt to put some money in the bank and was working as a messenger with a law firm in Birmingham. Assigned to deliver legal documents, I made my way across town to the Tutwiler Hotel on a scorching-hot day with a package marked "urgent."

"Darling," the client purred as the door to her opulent suite swung open. "Come in. Come in. In that little envelope you are carrying the key to my prison cell."

Though temporarily blinded by the sun streaming through the large French windows, I could not help but notice that the dishwater blonde standing before me was an exotic woman with crushed ruby lips. She was wearing a flamboyant red peignoir and a lot of gold jewelry. She thrust a cold martini glass into my hand.

"Cheers," she said, clinking her glass against mine.

Until that moment, alcohol had never touched my lips. I grew up Baptist Christian in the Deep South in the 1940s and 1950s and had walked a path of born-again living and Bible study. I emerged at age twenty-one a rather self-righteous party-pooper. After my beloved Blanche had retired, my devotion had shifted to a new friend named Jesus. I foreswore alcohol in His name. I vowed never to tip a glass and had kept to my word.

Now I was draining the last drops of the forbidden fruit and asking for more. For the next twenty years, I couldn't get enough. No matter how many times I reached for a bottle, I heard a voice echoing in my head, "You ought to be ashamed of yourself. You'll never amount to anything. When are you going to straighten up and fly right?"

It was Momma's voice. She had divorced Daddy when I was nine years old. Although I like to think that she did so because he was abusive to his children, I suspect she had reasons of her own for ending the marriage. Life in our house was hard, with little income and many mouths to feed. Mother worked every day as a secretary and her hard life left her bitter, with precious little emotion to shower on my brothers and sisters and me. Not once do I remember Momma telling us that she loved us or that she was proud of anything we did. As far back as I can recall, each of us was an island, separate and starving for some encouragement.

I sought refuge in the happy endings of double features at the movies and got lifted higher than a kite on music played in church and on the radio. A chorus of the stir-'em-up gospel standard "Nearer My God to Thee" could rouse me to my feet much the same as a pop-chart hit like "Earth Angel." Art also lifted me up. When our elementary school class visited the museum, I would practically walk into the large splashy paintings on display.

Looking back, I believe my sensitivity was leading me into a life of escape, which was taking shape in my mind, where I would play make-believe games. When I was a small child, for instance, I began assigning gender designations to colors and numbers, deciding that red was male and yellow was female, while four and five were boys and three was a girl. I believed in Santa Claus longer than most kids and hoped that a guardian angel would rescue me from the horrors of real life. These horrors included my father's behavior, my family's poverty, and especially my clubfeet.

The period from 1957 until 1979 is something of a blur for me. Moving from Birmingham to New York, Atlanta to Mobile, Mobile to California, I never felt connected to anything. I never kept a job for very long. I worked in advertising, sold real estate and ladies ready-to-wear. By 1979, I was dead broke, unemployable, and living in a postage stamp–size apartment in Long Beach, California, driving a beat-up old clunker. In the quiet of my mind, I would sometimes drift back to the idyllic days I spent in church memorizing the scriptures. One verse often reverberated in my head. "What does the Lord require of thee, but to do justly, and to love mercy and to walk humbly with thy God?"

"Who was God, anyway?" I wondered. Little did I know at the time, it was only when I hit bottom and was ready to confront my alcoholism some months later that I began to hear that voice.

# CHAPTER 4

# Turning Up the Volume

I DRANK MY LAST DROP OF ALCOHOL on February 17, 1980.

After more than twenty years of destructive carousing, my epiphany came when I was arrested for drunk driving. When those whirling blue lights signaled for me to pull over, I knew that the gig was up. It wasn't the first time I'd been thrown in jail for drinking and driving, but something inside of me knew, somehow, it would be the last.

Riding in the squad car, barreling down the back streets of Long Beach in the wee hours of the morning, I heard a voice in my head say, "It's over." Now, I am not one to hear voices and have always taken the magic of New Age spirituality with a healthy dose of skepticism. Still, I knew something special was happening. It was not just the thought that had startled me, it was the accompanying serenity that came upon me. Sitting in a police car, which was the most stressful experience I have ever had, I felt a tremendous calm. Yes, it *is* over, I thought to myself. I could feel it. Within a week, I had signed up for a drunk-driving diversion program.

Going from being a drunk to being a teetotaler was a long process fueled by waves of intuition. For me, it began each morning when I would lie in bed trying to receive more inspiration, which is what I called the voice I had heard after being arrested. More real than anything I had ever experienced in Sunday School, the voice reminded me of what Blanche had described—the murmur of angels. I was hungry to have that tingling feeling again. So I began to dedicate time each morning to listening, in case God had something to say. As I looked back on my life, I realized that I had talked to God often. That's what praying was. But I never paused even for a second to give Him a chance to answer back.

In the beginning very little happened. I was quiet and I did the best I could to still my mind, trying to appreciate the meditative quality of the experience. Sometimes my lips would tremble or I would get goose bumps whenever I thought I heard something. But I was cautious. The last thing I wanted was to fool myself.

Then one day, most certainly, I heard the voice in my head again and the message was clear and strong: "Ego is enemy."

Ego? I wondered. Whose ego? And what is ego, anyway? In my own understanding of the word, the ego was how I interacted with the world to satisfy my own desires. Sometimes my ego served me well. It helped me make my way in the world in a fair and conscientious way. But for most of my adult life my ego had gotten way out of control. And those were the times I got into trouble, big trouble.

Shortly after hearing these words, I began to write an inventory. I wanted to know exactly how my ego had gotten out of bounds. One day I even made a list of my flaws. Here's how it looked:

## Albert's Negative Points

1. Called other people hypocrites while ignoring my own faults.
2. Cheated on exams.
3. Stole what my parents wouldn't buy me.

4. Thought I was better than everyone else.

5. Was contemptuous of others prior to investigation.

6. Lied, even when the truth would have sufficed.

7. Drank to excess, ate to excess, and accumulated credit card debt.

There they were. My seven deadly sins. As I stared down at the list, I needed a minute to catch my breath. Who was this dastardly fellow, rotten to the core, with little to redeem him? Who was this man, causing so much static he could barely hear himself think?

I have always been a fan of Joseph Campbell, a transpersonal psychologist and author, who, according to the Joseph Campbell Foundation, was very influenced by the psychological studies of Freud and Jung, the art of Picasso and Henri Matisse, and the novels of Henry James and Thomas Mann. Thinking about ego, I recalled how Joseph Campbell had touched on the subject in his mythological version of how the earth was created. In *The Power of Myth*, Campbell describes the rebellion of Lucifer and his minions, how they left paradise and set up camp on earth, which God set aside for these outcasts. To stay in the Order of Lucifer, fallen angels took a vow never to say the name of God. Campbell contended that all of us are fallen angels, separated from God by lawless egos, and that our redemption can only come by speaking to God directly and learning to make better choices.

Looking back at my own life, I had to admit that despite all of my conventional religious training I never really felt connected to God. Quite the opposite. Very often I was lonely and afraid, going back to the time I was a little boy. If I had to be honest with myself, I'd admit fear was the principle emotion that drove me. Much like Edgar Bergen's dummy, Charlie McCarthy, I had been doing what my ego drove me to do out of some misguided idea that this would bring peace and control. In the absence of true spirituality, my ego had taken charge of me, helping to create a life of illusion and deception woven around addictions. The authentic me, the child of God, had been pushed to the background.

This was an interesting paradox to me. A healthy ego is important not only to survive but also to flourish in the world, but it can sabotage. I understood I needed to rein my ego in, but how? And then it dawned on me; like two kids whose ankles are tied together in a foot race, my ego and I must cooperate, work together to find a balance. As this thought crossed my mind, I remembered a verse I had learned as a boy at church: "Out of the depths I cry to thee, Lord hear my prayer, let thine ears be attended to the voice of thy supplicant." I would cry out and then I would listen. And what I would hear would guide me.

CHAPTER 5

# Forgiveness Is the Path to Clearing

ALL OF MY LIFE I had been told that God loved me. Dedicated now
to improving myself, I felt it was truly so. God seemed to be enticing
me to reconcile with Him in a language I had never before spoken or
understood. Each day, as if by magic, I found myself guided by messages and directions carried by people and coincidences, as well as
synchronicities and intuitions. If I followed a hunch and turned on
the radio, the announcer's advice seemed especially relevant to me.
On several occasions I found my way to books by authors who spoke
directly to my concerns.

That was the case with Emmet Fox, a popular spiritualist and
metaphysician in the 1930s who wrote ten books that sold more
than ten million copies. Fox had many illuminating things to say, but
one idea in particular struck a chord with me. As Fox put it, "To
refuse to forgive oneself is spiritual pride. 'And by that sin fell the
angel.' "

In his book *The Power of Constructive Thinking,* Fox extols the
Lord's Prayer as perhaps the single most important prayer in the
whole of Christianity because of its link to forgiveness. "The Lord's
Prayer issues general amnesty to those who beseech God," Fox

states. "The forgiveness of others is the vestibule of heaven. You have to get rid of all resentments and condemnations of others, and not least, of self-condemnation and remorse."

This felt like a very critical piece of the puzzle that I was trying to solve, offering a way out of my egocentric past. Fox suggested that the failure to forgive allows resentments to build up, which keeps us mired in guilt and attached to those who we perceive to be our enemies. Fox saw these attachments as keeping us shackled to the ones we hate. Until we forgive and release them and ourselves, other people with the same odious traits will keep coming into our lives until we face what lessons we need to learn. The path to freedom is forgiving others and ourselves.

## The Lord's Prayer

*Our Father who art in heaven, Hallowed be thy name.*
*Thy kingdom come. Thy will be done on earth, as it is in heaven.*
*Give us this day our daily bread.*
*And forgive us our debts, as we forgive our debtors.*
*And lead us not into temptation, but deliver us from evil:*
*For thine is the kingdom, and the power, and the glory, forever.*
*   Amen.*
*For if ye forgive men their trespasses, your heavenly Father will*
*   also forgive you:*
*But if ye forgive not men their trespasses, neither will your Father*
*   forgive your trespasses.*

Reading the prayer really opened my eyes. Due to my long history of drinking, I had harmed many people whose forgiveness I had not sought. And I harbored resentments toward others. If unforgiveness was the static we must clear in order to speak to God and hear His answers, I had work to do. I needed to come to terms with myself.

Having brought Albert's negative points to the surface (see page 20), I decided to try to love myself and embrace my ego rather than labeling it evil and trying to annihilate it. I did so in a forgiveness letter addressed to myself, which went like this:

Dear Albert:

I am writing you this amends letter to free us both from self-pity and from being victims. I will not say, "I'm sorry," or that "I apologize" for my part in the bruised feelings with family and friends. Most of us have been using such empty and meaningless expressions all our lives to wiggle away from true absolution. In order to seek forgiveness from you I am going to change.

I never allowed you to accept yourself. You were born with clubfeet and short of stature, and I said, "God should have made you a perfect specimen of a man." Remember how you loved the biblical story of Jesus inviting Zacchias to come down from the tree so that they could eat together? Zacchias had gone up the tree because he was short and wanted to be able to see Jesus. Jesus loved Zacchias no matter his height, but I would not let you identify with this love.

You were born into financial privation and I made you believe that you had been switched at birth, like the prince and the pauper. "You don't need to get along with the Gauldens," I whispered. I made you supersensitive about every word and every glance from everybody all of your life. "You need to divide and conquer friends" was a coaching ploy from me. Hence, your passive-aggressive behavior made people furious with you.

You cheated on exams when you knew the answers because I made you doubt yourself. You stole things you didn't need or want because I nudged you. Ice cream and candy and finally too much booze were my weapons to keep you attached to my godless ways. I sprinkled in fear and anger, with resentment toward those who took away what you thought was yours or were not going to give you what you wanted.

What I never counted on was that you would one day get quiet enough to hear God when He spoke to you.

I ask you to forgive me and would like us to form an alliance. As twin souls, let's embrace whatever principles we need to be precious children of God.

I love you and I honor you,
Your ego-self

My next biggest challenge was asking forgiveness from the one I perceived to have been my true enemy: my mother. I wrote this letter in 1980.

Dear Mother:

You know that I have struggled with my feelings about you and me since I was a youngster. I thought you were tough and I always wanted you to love me and I don't think that you ever have. Throughout my childhood, more than anything, I wanted you to take joy in who I was and what I accomplished. I never felt that you did, until my perceptions of what happened changed.

Mother, please forgive me for being angry with you because you didn't show up when I won the spelling bee, or read a poem in the city-wide contest, or was in a play or tapped into the National Honor Society. Someone pointed out to me that you were a single mother working five and a half days a week to support six children. You were doing what you had to do. I saw you as a martyr when I should have seen you as a caring mother.

I accused you of being ashamed of me when in truth I

did not accept myself. Blaming you for my clubfeet and being short has nearly destroyed me. When I labeled you self-righteous, I was describing my own worst defect of character. I was the drunk, not you. You cosigned loans and I never paid them because I was trying to get back at you. Now I know that the circumstance God created for me was my opportunity to succeed with God's continuing guidance. But I left God and you in my wake.

I ask you to forgive me for how I harmed you. My amends will be to treat my life as God's business, not mine. When I see a chance to do for someone else I will, in your name.

I have a picture of you on my desk. When I look at it I whisper, "I love you, Mom."

Please forgive me,
Albert

After writing to my mother, I made a list of all the other people I had hurt. This list included friends, family members, business associates, and acquaintances. Some were dead and I didn't know how to reach others to make amends. But I reached out to all I could.

This act of humility—asking others to forgive me for my transgressions—was the most healing thing I had ever done. I felt it was an elixir that set me free to start my life over. It helped me to see clear to the next stepping-stone on my path.

CHAPTER 6

# Through the Looking Glass

I HAD WORKED ON FORGIVING MYSELF and I had sought forgiveness from those whom I had harmed. The final step of my true emancipation came from seeing the value in what happened to me as a child. Like Alice from *Alice in Wonderland* after she passed through the looking glass, I discovered a whole new reality when I took a close look at my parents—who they were and how they had influenced me. My qualities as a person were clearly a combination of my mother's and father's negative and positive aspects. Examining the two people who raised me was imperative. I began with my father.

| *Father's Character Defects* | *Father's Good Qualities* |
|---|---|
| 1. Alcoholic | 1. Sense of humor |
| 2. Physically abusive to my mother | 2. High energy |
| 3. Emotionally abusive to me | 3. Inspired me |
| 4. Financially irresponsible | 4. Good friend |
| 5. Passive-aggressive | 5. Helped others |

6. Lazy

7. Narcissistic

8. Lying

9. Cheating

10. Abandoned his six children

6. Founded Little Boys' Baseball

And I continued on to my mother.

| Mother's Character Defects | Mother's Good Qualities |
| --- | --- |
| 1. Self-righteousness | 1. Good provider |
| 2. Overly critical | 2. Good moral example |
| 3. Judgmental | 3. Disciplinarian |
| 4. Too analytical | 4. Intelligent |
| 5. Never showing love | 5. Beautiful |
| 6. Didn't protect me from abuse | 6. Independent |

In looking over the list, I noticed that the positive and unattractive qualities that I shared with my parents were many.

From my father I inherited:

| Father's Character Defects | Father's Good Qualities |
| --- | --- |
| 1. Alcoholic | 1. Sense of humor |
| 2. Financially irresponsible | 2. High energy |
| 3. Passive-aggressive | 3. Good friend |
| 4. Lying | 4. Helped others |
| 5. Cheating | |

And from my mother I inherited:

| Mother's Character Defects | Mother's Good Qualities |
|---|---|
| 1. Self-righteousness | 1. Good moral example |
| 2. Overly critical | 2. Intelligent |
| 3. Judgmental | 3. Independent |
| 4. Too analytical | |

## Father's Story

My father was from a poor Irish family from North Carolina. Like generations of men before him in the bloodline, my daddy drank and lived beyond his means. His extravagances were legendary. Although Momma had a tough time feeding and clothing her kids, Daddy would come home with expensive toys for my sister Mary and my brother Bill—forgetting my brother Hank and me— or oftentimes, a fancy dress or gold earrings for our momma.

All of his defects infected me. I drank. I had married and divorced in a blackout. I often bought expensive gifts or flew away to exciting vacations instead of making my house payment.

Like Daddy, I was a liar. When I was seven or eight years old I remember scribbling in my older sister's textbook. When Daddy lined me and my siblings up for interrogation, I outright lied when he asked who marked up the book. Lacking a confession, he punished all of us. When he got ready to belt me he whispered, "I know you didn't do it, so I'll just lightly tap you."

Daddy taught me a motto: "Laugh and the world laughs with you; cry and you cry alone." On the gloomiest day, Daddy could find something to celebrate—if he was in the right mood. If he wasn't, a bright sun and blue sky could turn to black when his dark side engaged. He would slap at his kids and hit Momma.

He would often show up hours late—a classic passive-aggressive ploy. Or he would tell Momma that he'd eat whatever she had fixed for supper and then complain that he wanted something else. His narcissism demanded he occupy center stage when he was home. It was all about him, even when he arrived home after being gone for days with a mistress. He would brush off his absence with a lie that he had to work triple shifts at Tennessee Coal and Iron, where he was employed, and return to life as usual.

I had not seen my father since 1965. Around the time I was defining him in order to clear myself, my siblings had been telling me he was not well. He was blind and suffering from congestive heart failure. It took a little courage, but I wrote to him. In my letter I talked about how much I missed him and that I was sad that silent scorn had robbed me of knowing him better.

He called me on the phone a week later and told me how much he loved me. He said that he was happy that I had made something of my life. "I was so glad that you were not a jock like me and your brothers. When you were born with clubfeet, some part of me rejoiced thinking that you might become a teacher or a writer—really affect people's lives. Sports entertain for a night; a book can touch the world for years and years."

When we hung up the phone, I reassessed his life and mine for hours, as my impression all those years had been that he was a self-ish, egotistical, and drunken womanizer. I was trying to make room for the man who he had become, the man, he told me, who was now sober and married to the same woman for many years. The crusty cover protecting my heart from the pain of never having had a true relationship with my father began to soften, and I was able to make peace with him. I let him in where once he had been locked out of my thoughts and feelings.

My sister Margie called me at five o'clock the next morning to tell me that Daddy was dead.

## Mother's Story

Since my dad was out of the house from the time I was nine years old, it was Mother whose negative traits loomed larger. She complained about everything and could judge and criticize a person or situation to distraction. My room was never clean enough; I didn't do the dishes right or broke too many while drying them. Mother never complimented me for good grades or any honors I won. She felt that praise for these things was unnecessary. There was a joke among my brothers and sisters and me that we needed to ply mother with strong coffee or she would stay grouchy all day. How could coffee alter her attitude? I had no clue, but she could be rosy and funny after two cups.

Momma's inability to nurture and hug us was astounding to me until I realized that I too keep most people at a distance. Despite intense inner work, intimacy is still hard for me. I mask it with a friendly, affable exterior, but I distrust myself in relationships so much that I plot their ending before they get a good start.

I learned from my mother to become best friends with the most popular kid in class and to win acceptance by proxy. From kindergarten through high school I insinuated myself in the good graces of teachers. I was so needy that I had to be number one with whoever was my mentor that term. College was a rude awakening, for I wasn't able to charm or cajole my professors. I was graded on what was on the paper. Hence, I left college early.

The turning point in my relationship with my mother came right after my father died. Although I had tried to get closer to her after I stopped drinking, intimacy was hard for both of us. But we both kept making attempts to meet in the middle. While having lunch one day, she told me something that cleared up a lifetime of resentment toward her.

"Albert, did you know that my mother died when I was six years old?"

My mother went on to explain how her father relied on her brothers and sisters to look after her, as he had to work every day as an engineer. As she recounted her childhood, it became apparent to me that she had done the best she could as a mother when she had never really had one of her own.

We stayed longer at the restaurant than usual that day because we both knew we needed to get to know each other better. We laughed until we cried, and we swapped stories about our critical, judgmental ways and came to see that we were mirrors of each other.

When we were finished, I said to her, "Mother, you have truly been my best teacher."

## Seeing the Lessons Clearly

Examining my parents not only revealed their defects, it also showed me what I needed to overcome in myself. One's natural God-given abilities can surface when our fears and insecurities are faced. Unmasking and stopping pretense can open the door for unlimited successes. Identifying with another's problems and difficulties humanizes our relationships. Controlling everything and everybody causes others to be repelled and flee. The more I trusted God and turned to Him for guidance, the less I tried to steer.

God, as father and mother, began to heal what formerly divided me within myself. As I practiced hearing what He said to me and going where he led, I felt my life getting better and better.

# CHAPTER 7

# Starting Over

SOON AFTER I CLEARED UP MY PAST with my parents, it became quite evident that I was changing in a fundamental way. It is not an exaggeration to say that I felt I was being reborn. God was using a language of signs, symbols, and synchronicities to help me remake my life, and I was doing the footwork. Thought impressions, intuitions, and hunches came often. I felt I were being led to a life of higher purpose. Yet a burning question remained: What else must I do and what must I continue to do to fulfill my higher purpose?

One simple technique I tried was writing this question on a piece of paper each night and falling asleep with it under my pillow. Some nights I got messages in dreams that solved some of the rebirth puzzle. Over time I came up with the following list:

1. Stay attuned to God through prayer and meditation

2. Seek forgiveness from those I had harmed

3. Change playgrounds and playmates

4. Make restitution for financial wrongs

5. Think and speak positive thoughts

6. Try to be of service to others

7. Most important: Watch for signposts from God

After I had worked with dreams for a while, I began to see signs of God's direction for my life and to act upon them. Before I got sober I had been in a local motivational speakers group with a man who now attended the same daily recovery meetings I did. One day he asked me if I could apply some of the principles of sobriety and speak to a group of salespeople in his company at their annual convention. I knew in my gut that this was another of God's opportunities, so I accepted his offer. The topic was "Change to Make Your Life Better."

As I stood before more than 200 men and women, I spoke without notes. What I told the group was that I wouldn't change anything—not near bankruptcy, nor the drunk-driving arrest or loss of credit standing, not even all the amends I had to make for the harm I had caused many people. It felt good to speak from my heart and not to try to razzle-dazzle the audience. The man who hired me to speak told me later that it was refreshing to hear someone talk to a crowd without a self-serving ego holding court.

"To change one thing would mean that everything else would not be the same," I said. "I am so much happier today than I was a year or more ago, or even than I have ever been before. I am free from living a life of blind ambition. I try to live with honesty and purpose, where success at any price once trapped me on a dead-end street. Today when I run into you on the street, I don't hide my head. When I get a letter from a bank or an attorney, I open it as I would a letter from a friend. If I buy it, I pay for it on time. I have a different power driver than I used to have."

A thirty-something gentleman came up to me after the meeting and asked me if I had had a religious experience. I told him that I preferred to think of it as having become quiet enough to hear God's voice and to see his hand at work in what I now thought of as the new language.

"How do you do that?" he asked.

We went for coffee and I told him what had happened to me. He promised to let me know what had happened to him after the getting-quiet period. Although it did not occur to me then, I had just unofficially counseled my first student.

## Teaching Others the New Language

My life took another big shift in 1981 when a middle-aged woman asked me if I would counsel her. She had heard me speak in recovery meetings and told me that I had something that she wanted.

"What exactly is that?" I asked.

"Honesty," she replied. "You are very open about having made a lot of mistakes, which you called touchstones. I am ready for a flawed therapist."

I decided to take a leap of faith and work with her. She began coming to see me once a week and soon her two daughters signed on. Their friends came along next. Through word of mouth, my counseling practice was achieving liftoff. I had obtained credentials through an association of alternative therapists, and my client base grew as one person told another about the results of our work.

Around my second year of sobriety, while I was still living in California, a series of events seemed to be setting up a chain reaction in my life. One of my new clients had a sister who was a producer and host of a morning show in Seattle. The producer asked me to fly up and do a segment on personal-growth counseling. A bookstore owner from Phoenix who was visiting there saw me on the show and invited me to do a workshop in Arizona. On a day trip to Sedona, a community about 100 miles north of Phoenix, the day before I returned to California, I had a mystical feeling. I was drawn to move there. When I got back to Long Beach, I saw a large piece of paper tacked to my door. Upon closer inspection, I found that it was an eviction notice. I had failed to sign my new lease within the designated time. I took this as a sign that God wanted me in Sedona.

My life, which had been upside down for so long, fell quickly into place. In 1986, the Sedona Intensive was born, featuring a licensed psychologist, massage therapists, network chiropractors, and a transformational breath worker, as well as other practitioners and me. Thanks to hunches and intuitive road maps along the way, my life purpose was emerging. God was taking a flawed man and letting him share his journey of healing with others.

Two men who affected my life at this time stand out. The first was Joseph Campbell, author of *The Power of Myth,* whose work was instrumental in pushing me to look for the "central mystery of my experience." Campbell wrote that "if you don't know what the guide-signs are along the way, you have to work it out for yourself." He spoke of shutting out the distractions that keep us from the magic of self-creation.

The second great influence was Paulo Coelho, Brazilian author of *The Alchemist,* which has been published in more than forty languages and sold more than twenty-three million copies worldwide. *The Alchemist* is an allegory about a young shepherd named Santiago from Spain who follows his dream of treasure all the way to the pyramids in Egypt. The young boy is told that "when you want something, all the universe conspires in helping you to achieve it."

What clicked for me in Coelho's book were the words of the king who tells the young seeker Santiago that "there is a language in the world that everyone understands, but has forgotten; a language without words . . . and about omens." The shepherd boy later says that he is searching for that universal language.

Santiago's experience had been my own quest. I had been diving into a strong current that carried me to counsel others. As I did, hunches and intuitions and signposts led me. Clearly they were part of a divine language that time and diversions had caused me to forget—a language that would reconnect and guide me and others. I wanted to help others come alive to this universal language, which could lead to true identity and rebirth for all of us. "When you really want something, it's because that desire originated in the soul of the universe," writes Coelho. "It's your mission on earth."

I had known this truth and felt it. In some ways, my life had paralleled that of the shepherd. I had been roaming the world following my own personal legend, and I had had many omens. Signs from God had gotten me to where I was. There was a current, a flow, and I was being swept along on it. God was whispering about it in my ear, and I was learning to listen to God's mother tongue. I called it the new language, though it was primordial, as old as time and humanity. And I set about resurrecting it for others.

# PART II

# Breaking through to the New Language

CHAPTER 8

# Defining the New Language

WHEN I FIRST BEGAN to listen and look for God's signals, I had a rough time. This was uncharted territory for me, and I didn't know what I was supposed to be listening *to* or looking *for*. How could I trust what I heard and saw without having had any experience with all the ways God might be trying to speak to me? Discernment was important because I wanted to make a smart choice between God's will and wishful thinking.

One thing that I did was to continue to pray and meditate. I figured if I wanted to walk the path God had laid down for me and to hear Him when He spoke, I had better use the tools He had given me. As I began to sharpen my ability to recognize the difference between God's will and self-will, I realized that it would be helpful to define the phenomena that I had been experiencing.

I am going to outline what I discovered about the new language, how it is spoken and heard, in the following Glossary of the New Language. I have attempted to be comprehensive, including all the methods God uses as He guides and steers us.

## A Glossary of the New Language

### Acts of Nature

In biblical times, God often spoke through acts of nature. A rainbow was a sign of God's covenant, or promise, to Noah. A burning bush was a visible manifestation of God Himself to Moses. And a gust of wind was used in Genesis as a sign of the force of creation. When the suffering Job asked God to explain his travails, the Lord answered Job "out of the whirlwind," which was a frequent sign of theophanies, or divine appearances, in the ancient times. God still speaks to us today through natural occurrences of all sorts. The wind, rainstorms, clouds, fire, and rainbows can all carry divine messages.

*Example:* I once walked out of an art exhibition alongside the artist being featured, and we both saw a rainbow arched over the gallery. Without hesitation, the artist said, "There's my sign that my show will sell out." It did.

*Example:* A client of mine named Howell takes long walks when he is contemplating a problem. As remedies float through his head, often a sudden gust of wind knocks him down even on a relatively still night. He finds the wind a confirmation that he is on the right track in his search for solutions. Events have proven his theory correct.

### Angel Murmur

An angel is a spiritual being superior to man who serves as a messenger from God. A murmur is a soft or gentle utterance. An angel murmur is God's way of making contact with us through a soft voice in our ear when we need special or urgent help or advice.

*Example:* Jonathan, who is a client of mine, was driving to a meeting out of town when he distinctly heard a voice whisper, "Go home." The voice repeated the command three times in a short period of time. Jonathan turned the car around and when he arrived home he found that his wife was sick and needed to go to the hospital.

### Cautions

A sudden or dramatic warning or admonishment that may come as a gut feeling, an intuition, or as a physical obstacle is a caution. A caution may also come as a whisper in our ear or a thought impression in our head that feels unmistakably like an idea not our own.

*Example:* My friend Will was supposed to catch a six o'clock flight out of Dallas–Fort Worth airport. He felt a strong urge to catch the seven-thirty flight instead and changed his plan, though he was at risk of missing his meeting. The six o'clock flight crashed upon takeoff.

*Example:* Mary was trying to make hotel reservations to visit Perugia, Italy, in September of 1997. Every time she tried to reach her travel agent the phone would go dead. After a couple of days of not being able to reach anyone, Mary had the strongest thought impression that she should not go at all. She could see the Basilica of Saint Francesco in Assisi the next spring. The day she was to have arrived, there was an earthquake that did severe damage to the basilica and its convent.

### Click

A click is a sound that represents two pieces that belong together or lock together, like a seat belt engaging, or a key turning in a lock. When two people find they have much in common, they are said to click. If an event goes off without a hitch, this is also known as clicking. It is as if divine Providence had drawn people together for a purpose and they find a magnetic unison.

*Example:* When Sally walked into a large convention center where computer technology was being demonstrated, she felt drawn to a particular exhibitor and struck up a conversation with her. Within months, they became business partners.

### Coincidence

When events seem to have some connection without an apparent plan or design, this is coincidence. This is one of the most recognizable of all manifestations of God operating on invisible planes. Each individual is an energy force field and time-to-meet messages are sent along gridlines in our nervous system.

*Examples:* Santiago, a Sedona Intensive graduate, had recently arrived in Miami from Colombia and needed a place to live. Silvia wanted to rent a room in her house after her husband died. Santiago and Silvia sat at the counter next to each other in a restaurant and struck up a conversation. That day Santiago rented a room in Silvia's house.

### Daydream

A daydream is a visionary, usually wishful, creation of the imagination. Combined with meditation, daydreams can provide insights into God's will for one's life.

*Example:* Art sat at his desk at work in his suit and tie and frequently daydreamed about working on the beaches of Maui in his swimsuit. Daydreams led to meditating about living and working in Hawaii. Before long he was transferred by the company to the field office in Kapalua.

### Dreams

A dream is a series of thoughts, images, or emotions occurring during sleep—a visionary creation of the imagination. God often speaks in our dreams. As a form of premonition, a dream can foretell the future or provide a pictorial sounding board for problems soon to be encountered.

*Example:* A friend of mine, Alexander, couldn't decide where to go on vacation. He was thinking about several possibilities as he fell asleep. He had a vivid dream about blue waters with blindingly white houses on a mountaintop. The next morning he was leafing through travel brochures when he saw Mykonos—the Jewel of the Greek Isles—splashed across a photograph that was exactly as he had seen in his dreams. He booked his trip and had a fabulous time.

### Echo Effect

This is God's use of repetition of events, ideas, or people to make a point. God is underlining what cannot be ignored. The echo effect is the experience of hearing the same thing or seeing the same people or object or message in a short span of time.

*Example:* A client of mine named Sasha couldn't decide between a job offer in Dallas and one in San Francisco. She asked each morning in prayer and meditation for help in making the right decision, between two equally good choices. The day she had to make a decision she picked up a magazine that featured a story about life in San Francisco. She also happened to see a television in a storefront that had a baseball game featuring the San Francisco Giants. Interesting, she mused, as she turned on the radio to hear Tony Bennett singing "I Left My Heart in San Francisco." Sasha heeded the echoing signs she was receiving and took the job in San Francisco.

### Epiphany

An epiphany is a sudden manifestation or perception of the essential nature or meaning of something. It is an intuitive grasp of reality through something usually simple but striking.

*Example:* Warren wrote me that he had had such deep business problems that he had decided to leave his family and his financial difficulties behind him. As he packed to leave he was watching a woman on television. "You may not believe in you, but God does," she said. Struck by her words of encouragement, Warren called his minister for help. He stayed with his family and his business soon turned around.

## Foreshadowing

When one event heralds another and prepares us for a culminating occurrence, that is foreshadowing.

*Example:* Muriel, a client for many years who lives in Chicago, was convinced that she had seen her sister, Margaret, three times on the same day. A short time later, Margaret made an unexpected visit to Muriel's from Des Moines, delivering news that would affect Muriel's financial future.

## God-by-Proxy

The principle that God speaks to us through other people is the underpinning of the meaning of God-by-proxy. God uses the people in our life to get our attention and get His message and guidance across.

*Example:* My friend Mike was worried about how his daughter was going to spend her year off from college. At a business lunch with six men whom he had never met, one happened to mention that his wife counseled students taking time off from college. Mike, who never knew such counselors existed, got her card and followed up.

## Gut Reaction

A gut reaction is an intuitive response to a person or situation, which involves arousing basic emotions. It is an immediate response without forethought.

*Example:* A client's sister named Laurette was waiting for an elevator in the building where she worked. When the door opened, something told her not to get in. "I forgot something in my office," she said and turned away. Later she found out that someone had been raped that night in one of the elevators. Her gut instinct perhaps saved her from an attack.

*Example:* As soon as my friend's husband walked into his hotel room in Atlanta, he got a gut feeling to go out into the hall to check to see where the fire exit was. That night he was awakened by a fire alarm. The kitchen had caught fire, and he was quickly able to find his way to safety.

## Hunch

A hunch is a strong intuitive feeling concerning a future event or result.

*Example:* Ethel had a hunch that her neighbor Hans was ready to sell the five acres that separated their houses. She waved him over to her yard and asked him if he wanted to sell the acreage.

"Funny you should ask me today because my accountant just called five minutes ago and said it was time to sell."

## Inner Knowing

When you have no facts to back you up but some compelling urge or sense of understanding tells you what you know to be true, you are relying on your inner knowing. Although you must use cold reasoning to protect against making foolish choices, you also must always be true to yourself and your inner knowledge.

*Example:* When I was a little boy, everybody told Miss Towles that she was being foolhardy to stand up for my classmate Billy, but she kept her resolve. She knew he was a good person and could make something of himself.

"He's trailer trash. Look at those tattoos," said one teacher.

"He'll never amount to a hill of beans," said another.

In fits and starts Miss Towles tutored Billy; she disciplined him when he needed it and gave him lots of praise when it was deserved. Ten years later, Billy graduated first in his class at Princeton and made something of his life because of a teacher who believed in him.

### Intuition

Intuition is the power or faculty of attaining direct knowledge or cognition without the use of rational thought and factual information. It can also be referred to as quick-and-ready insight.

*Example:* Two friends, Giselle and Harriet, met for their usual Tuesday lunch.

"Do I have news for you!" said Giselle.

"You just got a big promotion," replied Harriet.

"Who told you?" asked Giselle.

"No one. It's woman's intuition, that's all," said Harriet.

### Omen

An omen is an occurrence or phenomenon believed to portend a future event.

*Example:* Ken was considering starting his own business, but fear held him back. However, every time he started thinking about the pros and cons of such a venture, a blue bird would fly onto a limb of his big oak tree. He dismissed the appearances of the birds as meaningless coincidence until the day he was sitting in his lawyer's office about to discuss the matter. At that moment he heard a strange sound at the window—it was another blue bird. Ken took the plunge, started his own company, and was very successful.

*Example:* Trent went for a job interview to be president of a large telecommunications company. As he pulled up to the curb at the building where the firm was located, a large black bird swooped toward him as if on a mission to do him harm. The chairman of the board, who was dressed all in black, greeted him with a frown, reminding Trent of the bird who tried to attack him. Trent decided not to take the job. Three weeks later the company filed for bankruptcy protection.

### Premonition

The anticipation of an event without conscious reasoning is a premonition. It is a notice or warning.

*Example:* As I finished my counseling session with a client, I had a premonition that she was suicidal. The words came out of my mouth without forethought, "Alexis, do you have a gun in your purse?"

Alexis did have a gun in her purse. She sat and talked about how desperate she was over her failed marriage and financial problems, and said she intended to end her life. As she talked, I was able to coax the gun from her.

### Ringing True

A fact rings true when you hear someone discussing something you know nothing about firsthand but a certain resonance and head-heart connection tells you that what you are hearing is true. The basis for this determination is divine, inborn intelligence.

*Example:* When Marcus heard his friend Maria talk about the benefit of spending a healing weekend in the Berkshires, he knew her pain had lifted. What she said rang true.

### Serendipity

Serendipity is the faculty of making fortunate discoveries by accident. Coined by British author Horace Walpole in a letter he wrote in 1754, the term "serendipity" was taken from a Persian fairy tale, *The Three Princes of Serendip:* "As their highnesses traveled they were always making by accident and discernment, of things which they were not in quest of."

*Example:* My client Vance traveled extensively throughout East

Asia not only for pleasure but to look for rare treasures for his import-export business. He had no method to his search but rather liked to walk along back streets. He swears that he stumbles across the best artifacts accidentally.

*Example:* I read an account in the *Phoenix Republic* about a woman named Aleda who was distraught that her cat had just died from old age. Grief stricken, she slipped into a church for solace. As she got up to leave she heard the meow of a cat. She followed the sound and found a Persian cat and her three kittens behind a set of stairs. The monsignor said that Aleda could have the cat and her litter.

## Signs

God gets His message across to us through billboards, postcards, business cards, headlines, and skywriting. Our attention may be caught through the unexpected but timely appearance of an animal, an object, or an event. Drama is often the flavor of the experience of receiving a sign, and it may carry advice or encouragement.

*Example:* My client Marilyn's life was a mess. She had not prepared her taxes, she was overdrawn on her checking account, and her house was disheveled. One morning, Marilyn's doorbell rang and there stood a deliveryman holding a package labeled "all-purpose cleaning detergent." It was addressed to her next-door neighbor, but Marilyn made no mistake—the message was for her.

*Example:* Terri heard from her boss that their company was downsizing and that she might be furloughed. On the same day her stockbroker called with bad news about her investments. Feeling low, she picked up *The New York Times* and headed to her favorite coffee shop for a latte. As she leafed through the pages of the newspaper, a headline caught her eye: ALL IS NOT LOST. Terri felt a twinge of hope.

### Synchronicity

The concept of synchronicity, discussed by Swiss psychologist Carl Jung, is used to describe meaningful coincidences. A synchronicity is a coincidence that always involves a crucial time element. An interaction between two people or parallel events without appointment or plan is synchronicity at work. Synchronistic experiences tend to be deeply personal—when a person sees in her own mind connections between her thoughts and objective events in the external world.

*Example:* Two old friends of mine shared this story with me: Two friends, Kate and Samantha, bumped into each other on the Via Veneto in Rome while they were both vacationing. They agreed to continue sightseeing together and unexpectedly stumbled onto an orphanage outside of Vatican City. Upon returning to the States, the friends nurtured a relationship with the Italian children from the orphanage and their caretakers. Five years later, Kate and Samantha underwrote a charity to help unwed Italian mothers get an education, obtain employment, and raise their babies rather than give them up for adoption.

### Telepathy

Telepathy is communication from one mind to another by extrasensory means. It's as if invisible telephone lines send messages between two or more people. Although this phenomenon amazes most of us, the accuracy of its relay has been scientifically documented. When one experiences telepathy, he or she is said to have ESP, extrasensory perception.

*Example:* I was writing a letter to a friend and just as I wrote, "Dear David," the telephone rang. David was on the phone and said my name had just popped into his head.

*Example:* A friend told me this story about his brother-in-law.

Dexter went to the store to buy groceries from his wife Charlotte's list. As he passed the laundry detergent section the idea popped into his head to buy all-purpose bleach. Putting away Dexter's purchases, Charlotte said, "Dexter, I can't believe you bought bleach. The minute I heard the car pull out of the drive, I wished I had put it on the shopping list. You must have ESP."

### Thought Impression

When a tutor of the mind seems to be giving you new ideas or altering your thinking but there is no audible sound, God may be speaking through thought impression. These thoughts are different from what you would take to be your own usual stream of consciousness. A thought impression may cause you to say, "Where did that idea come from?" Thought impressions are the ideas in your head that may not be your own.

*Example:* My client Stephen was so upset with his brother that he wanted to pick up the phone and blast him. He decided to rest in the hammock in his backyard to try to calm down before he made the call. Drifting in and out of a catnap, Stephen had strong thoughts that began to move him away from confrontation. He had a mental impression of how his brother had been through rough times with his son's problems at school and had lost customers due to a slowing economy. As he yawned and sat up he thought he heard the words in his head, "Love Bill, don't lash out at him."

*Example:* My friend Cindy had filled out an application in April to buy an extended health-care insurance policy for her husband, Bill. On October 29 of the same year, a thought kept popping into her head to send in the application with the check for the first premium. She did.

On November 4, Bill had a massive heart attack. They were saved from financial ruin because Cindy acted on a thought impression that wouldn't go away.

*Vision*

A vision is the mystical experience of seeing as if with the eyes of a supernatural being. The vision itself is usually a miraculous appearance that conveys a revelation.

*Example:* Nina and her friend Scott were standing at the window of her top-floor apartment in New York City about a quarter to nine one September morning. As Nina and Scott looked downtown at the World Trade Center, they saw an airplane plow into one of the towers. Moments later they saw a brilliant vortex and then a golden spiral staircase encircling the building with spirits ascending.

*Wonders*

This is God's use of awe and spectacle to bring attention to His omnipotence. It affirms the majesty of God's creativity and infinite power. It is the part of the language that cannot be strictly defined because it is open to such a wide variety of manifestations.

*Example:* I was stressed at the thought that the plans I had for the Sedona Intensive reunion were impossible. How could I possibly get 200 graduates to come back for a gathering at one time? No chance, I thought. Then my attention was drawn to the backdrop of Red Rock country: rust-red spires and craggy limestone mountains that were thousands of years old. I chuckled, "I can't do anything, but God can. I think I'll learn to let Him." The reunion took place and was a huge success.

*Example:* The director of the Summer Playhouse at the Hollywood Bowl woke up one Saturday morning to hear the weatherman forecast an 80 percent chance of rain. He was afraid the final soldout performance of his play would be washed out. Throughout the night lightning flashed and rain fell all around the Hollywood Bowl, but the downpour missed the people watching the performance.

CHAPTER 9

# Learning to Speak the New Language

NOW THAT WE HAVE DEFINED the new language, its texture and components, I want to show you how to recognize and use it in your everyday life. In order to do this, you must develop the art of appreciation that allows you to know what you hear when you listen and what you see when you look. If you don't develop these skills, you might wind up like the man in the classic story of the flood.

Sitting atop his house surrounded by rising water, the man prayed, "God, please help me." Soon a motorboat came to rescue him, but he refused to get in. Later a helicopter dropped a rescue ladder, but the man declined to climb up. When he drowned and went to heaven, he stormed up to Saint Peter and said, "I prayed for God's help and He did nothing."

"God sent a boat and helicopter," Saint Peter said. "Why did you refuse them?"

We have to know when God shows up. But how will His help come? As a motorboat? A helicopter? Let's consider some of the places you will find the new language at work.

In primitive times, when there was no mass media or technology, God seems to have worked through acts of nature, angel visitations, dreams, and voices. The ancient world was a quieter place with fewer distractions. And God may have had an easier time getting His message through to us. Today, in our multimedia environment, look to God to find us where our attention is.

## Newspapers and Magazines

Newspapers are loaded with messages straight from God's mouth. When I open up a newspaper, I skim the stories and the messages stand out in plain sight. Some people pore over each section, and they seem to find what they need. However quickly or slowly you peruse a newspaper or magazine, God's directions are scattered throughout.

Recently, I scanned a story in USA Today about a power outage in California. There was a picture of demonstrators holding picket signs that read: GIVE THE POWER BACK TO THE PEOPLE. While the power blackouts were a real problem in California, God was solving a business problem for me that morning, as I had been struggling with an uncooperative staff member. "Should I be sharing the power more than I am?" I wondered upon seeing the picket sign. The news story gave me pause—along with a lead to a solution. I often find that a story or advertisement may address whatever is on my mind at the time I'm reading a newspaper. I remain open because I know that this is one of the ways that God speaks to all of us.

How do I know what messages are for me? And how do I know the suggestions will work if they are for me? The process starts with what catches my attention. It has to do with developing a sense of knowing, which evolves with trial and error. Good judgment takes time to cultivate but the more I listen and learn to discern, the more my instincts prove to be right. And I believe that the truth has a special vibration that each of us can learn to feel. The truth in our ultrarational world has become a mere accumulation of facts and information. We are inundated by news twenty-four hours a day. But in the end, what do we know? God can cut through the information heap with a simple, profound bit of wisdom. The more we collaborate with Him, the better we become as a team. You might think about double partners in tennis who instinctively know where the other is going. My record for receiving accurate messages that help me in all areas of my life has improved with practice. And, at the very least, I get a sense of peace and calm because I believe God is ever present and that life is sacred.

## Movies, Television, and Plays

Powerful messages come to you through motion pictures, television, and stage plays. In order to decode the messages, you simply need to take note of what grabs you. God speaks to your heart. Track your feelings as a bounty hunter would his prey. Symbols can help you uncover rich meanings.

One day I was watching the movie *The Matrix*, which appeared to be a warp-speed, hi-tech motion picture about a computer game run amok—certainly there were no messages for me here. However, the main character was on a mission to find his true purpose in life, and I found myself becoming very involved in his quest, as I had just been talking to a friend about my own life's purpose. Through the exposition of the movie, I felt God was asking me to see if I was serving the purpose for which He had created me. Was there more that I could do? I felt God was clearly conversing with me, and I was eager to stay tuned for His guidance.

On another occasion, I was laughing with Niles and Frasier Crane of the hit television series *Frasier*, when I heard a plotline that spoke to me. Dr. Frasier Crane thought he was singing a few bars from an opera to a friend on the telephone, but he had been hoodwinked and was really singing live on his own radio station. When Frasier complained about the hoax, his friends told him to lighten up. Like the Frasier character, I had been taking myself way too seriously and that message spoke volumes to me. I felt a weight lifting from my shoulders with the laughter.

## Advertisements

Allison was stewing over an investment quandary when she opened the paper and saw an ad for a drip system that waters plants on a timer. It said, "You Don't Do a Thing." Allison didn't have any plants in her house, but she felt God was telling her to leave her portfolio alone.

I have gotten equally strong guidance from ads. Once I was concerned about paying off a sizable loan when I heard a woman on television say, "If you want your garden to grow, you better start planting Mrs. Adams Seeds today." The ad suggested an installment plan that would settle the loan in an orderly fashion. I took the advice and stopped worrying.

## Radio

Many clients report having heard God shots come over the radio. Sue told me that she didn't know what to do about her husband's infidelity when country singer Tammy Wynette told her to "Stand by Your Man." She felt the advice was worth a try, and they repaired their marriage. Oftentimes when I doubt myself about the Sedona Intensive, Frank Sinatra's "My Way" will come on the radio to give me courage to run it the way I see fit.

## Writing It Down

When I began listening and looking for the new language, I found it was helpful to keep a diary or a journal. You can do the same. Perhaps you will write in it each night or morning, or throughout the day. To help you illustrate how and where you will hear God through people, places, and things, I am going to open my journal to you.

## Day One, New Language Journal—July 27, 2001

7 A.M.—Hurriedly set out for Bell Rock vortex for my morning walk and saw a sign that said, PLEASE BE QUIET. MEDITATION GROUP UP AHEAD. I took this as a reminder to sit and meditate, which I did.

8 A.M.—I ate breakfast and read the paper. The first headline I saw said, ENERGY SLOWDOWN. I decided to eat more slowly and planned to conserve my energy today. I have been feeling overly tired.

9 A.M.—I was wondering whether or not to have my car washed. Out of nowhere the thought, It's going to rain, floated through my mind. I began my workday. An hour later rain began to pour down. I smiled at the warning I had.

10 A.M.—My printer jammed. I needed to print and send some letters to my secretary. Within three hours two of the letters were obsolete after phone calls from clients. I knew the printer wasn't working because the letters should not have been sent.

3 P.M.—Out of nowhere I started talking to a friend about mythology and Joseph Campbell. She said that she saw something in a catalog about his books being reprinted. I took a break to catch the news and the set was on PBS. Bill Moyers is talking to Joseph Campbell about *The Power of Myth*. Bingo! I had been struggling for days about a theme for an upcoming lecture. I sat down and wrote a flyer about language as myth.

7 P.M.—Sagan and I went to Dahl & DiLuca's Ristorante Italiano for dinner. A young woman named Carrie stopped by our table and introduced herself as the daugh-

ter of a good friend of mine. She told us that she was in Sedona for the summer and would like to get a job as a nanny. Two minutes before Carrie stopped at our table, Sagan told me that she needed help with her son for the month of August. Sagan and Carrie talked, and Sagan hired her.

For day one I indicated the new language I encountered and the message it had for me in bold. Day two I am going to let you figure out what events in my day were telling me.

## Day Two, New Language Journal—July 28, 2001

7:30 A.M.—I woke up and checked my E-mail and I had one message: Are you overweight? I went out to breakfast, and the manager of the restaurant asked me the name of the spa I go to every year.

"The Pritikin Longevity Center," I said.

"Have you been lately?" Bruce asked.

"No. Why do you want to know?"

"You always used to go in August or September."

My business partner, Scott, joined me for breakfast. He handed me the mail. I got a letter from the Pritikin offering me a twenty percent discount if I booked a week in August.

"Book me for two weeks beginning August 15," I said to Scott.

9:00 A.M.—I tried to write but found myself staring at a blank page. After twenty minutes, I went into the garden and lay down under the cottonwood trees and meditated. In a matter of minutes I got an idea to use the Internet to research my subject. The same three books were listed in the bibliography on all three sites. I glanced to my left where those three books lay on my table. I shut my eyes for a few seconds. Then I opened each book to certain pages. The pages I opened to in each book directly connected to what I was writing. For the next three hours I wrote without interruption.

1:00 P.M.—A friend called and asked me if I wanted to drive up to Flagstaff for an outdoor concert. I could use a break, I thought to myself. I had been writing all morning. Before I answered I looked at what I had just written: "No, I don't want to." The words rang true and I declined to go. That night my friend called to say that he had hit an elk on the drive up I-17 and had been in the emergency room for a couple of hours.

4:00 P.M.—I checked my private mailbox and had two letters. One was a solicitation from a credit card company and the other was a note from a client with a check for $2,000 enclosed. He said that he had owed me the money for more than ten years for work I had done when he needed help but was unable to pay.

7:00 P.M.—I decided to open a can of soup and make it an early night. I turned on the television and caught the start of the film classic *It's a Wonderful Life*.

## Arthur's Story

Through the years I have seen and heard thousands of examples of how the language works in the lives of my clients. Arthur Roberts, who lived in Los Angeles, had a remarkable series of God's flash cards in his life that brought him success in a real estate venture.

Arthur had been ill for several months. The first day he was able to go out of the house he ran into a friend named Fred he hadn't seen in years. During their conversation, Fred suggested that Arthur go to real estate school. And if Arthur would go to work for Fred, Fred would pay for the course to get Arthur's license. Arthur agreed to

Fred's terms because, just before running into Fred that day, Fred's business card had fallen out of a book Arthur had been reading.

The day his real estate license arrived, a friend stopped by Arthur's house and asked him to look at an estate 100 miles from the city that was about to go on the market. Although it seemed that the property was too far away for Arthur to show prospects, he went to look at the thirty-acre estate anyway. The minute he drove onto the property the owner, a woman named Elise Brown, came up to the car and asked Arthur if he was a realtor. He said that as of three hours ago he was. "I have a hunch you're going to sell this property," Mrs. Brown said.

The property was a one-of-a-kind manor and would appeal only to a special buyer. The estate was an hour from a major airport and was three miles off the highway down a dirt road. Arthur heard Mrs. Brown's words play in his head: "You're going to sell this property."

That night Arthur decided to try a new restaurant. He'd read about it in a magazine, and two friends said that it was not to be missed. He was seated next to a couple who were talking about looking for a house. The man kept insisting that it be on acreage and more remote. She wanted it to be on an unpaved road to discourage traffic. Arthur couldn't resist.

When he introduced himself, he discovered that the husband's name was also Arthur, Arthur Clayton. Mr. Clayton's wife, Sasha, had grown up near the property Arthur Roberts had just seen that day. When he began to tell them of the property, Sasha let out a gasp. "That property was a private Jesuit school I went to when I was a girl. I use to tell my friends I'd love to live there if the property was ever for sale."

The two Arthurs exchanged business cards.

"Look," said Mr. Clayton. "The last four digits of our telephone numbers are the same. And that accent of yours, where are you from?"

"I'm from Georgia," said Arthur.

"I was born in Georgia," said Mr. Clayton.

Early the next day the trio went to see the property, which the Claytons bought on the spot.

The new language spoke to Arthur five ways in a relatively short period of time:

1. Fred's business card falling from the book—**a sign**
2. Mrs. Brown's remark to Arthur Gold—**God-by-proxy**
3. Picking the restaurant—**echo effect**
4. Meeting the Claytons—**synchronicity**
5. Sasha Clayton had gone to school on the estate—**coincidence**

As an exercise to help you recognize when God is speaking to you in the new language, keep your own new-language journal for a few days. Then outline the various ways God is helping you make decisions, be more cautious, and listen when other people are speaking to you.

CHAPTER 10

# The Language of Coincidence

COINCIDENCE: A sequence of events or experiences that appear accidental while also seeming planned, prearranged, or closely related.

"At one time or another it's happened to all of us. There's that certain number that pops up wherever you go. Hotel rooms, airline terminals, street addresses—its haunting presence cannot be escaped. Or you're in your car, absently humming a song. You turn on the radio. A sudden chill prickles your spine. That same song is now pouring from the speaker," Peter A. Jordan writes in his book *The Mystery of Chance.* Then he asks, "Coincidence, or is it?"

The answer is yes. I agree with him that coincidences are "embedded in a higher, transcendental force, a cosmic 'glue' which binds random events together in a meaningful and coherent pattern." Perhaps, modern science would rather call these happenings an expression of chance—superstitions emerging from our imaginations. But many of us who use discernment in distinguishing divine strikes from wishful thinking refer to them as messages from God.

What is intriguing to me about Jordan's quote is that I had written something similar just prior to coming upon his book, but I liked the way he expressed his ideas better. Coincidentally, we were both on the same wavelength. The wavelength of coincidence is an important frequency in the new language, one of the ways God speaks to us.

In *Man and His Symbols*, Carl Jung writes that coincidences "are archetypes that become doorways that provide access to meaningful experiences." Coincidences, according to Jung, align with the notion that we live in a world that is united and interdependent and whose events emanate from one source. Historian Arthur Koestler's book *The Roots of Coincidence* relates coincidence to the "universal scheme of things."

Coincidences occur in the most routine parts of everyday life. Witness my client Debbie. Debbie was driving down the freeway in Southern California talking to her best friend, Meg. Debbie was asking Meg, "How do I make Edward understand what I want to say to him?" Just at that moment a car whose license plate read "BDEBBIE," cut in front of her truck. "Look," called out her friend, "interesting inscription."

Later Debbie had that talk with her boyfriend and things worked out because she spoke from her heart—she was herself. She may not ever have figured out what was appropriate to say to Edward if God had not intervened to help her.

Hundreds of clients tell me the same stories: While perusing the latest titles in a bookstore, a book that they were not looking for literally falls off the shelf. They buy it and it ends up changing their life. Or they have been pulled into a store while shopping and met someone significant, or overheard something that edified them or found something they had been looking for. I like to think that this is God reaching out to us with a sense of drama to catch our attention.

One cannot live his life waiting for coincidences to tell him what to do, but when they occur they are undeniable God shots.

They underline, italicize, and emphasize strong messages that we might otherwise ignore. Coincidences are events that take us out of the mundane and uneventful world in which we live and often thrust us into the eventful. Of course, we have to pay attention and value the coincidence for this to occur. And not everybody does. I know people who are inundated with coincidences, but they choose not to see them or act upon them. Those of us who live with our eyes wide open are more likely to heed what these messages are telling us.

When I was living in Mobile in 1970 I knew that my time there was limited, but I didn't know where to go next. For several days in a row I would see a car that had a bumper sticker that read, "California or bust."

If that person is supposed to go to California, I wondered, why are they still in Mobile? Staying on the lookout for the car and asking myself what I was going to do with my life, I turned on the radio and heard, "California Here I Come." That experience tipped the scale for me. A week later I quit my job at the advertising agency and headed for Los Angeles.

You may be thinking that it's just like a drunk to be on the move, but I believe that God is getting across to us, even when we don't want Him to. I believe that sign and that song were indications for me to go West, because California was where I learned a lot about myself and began to turn away from my bad habits.

## Client Stories

I believe that God uses coincidences to steer us on our path. Many examples from my clients confirm this.

Chip had signed up to take a civil-service examination in Colorado Springs to see if he qualified for training to become a policeman. When he got to city hall he found that he had misread the date for the exam—the test for the police force was to be administered the next month. Coincidentally, the test to see who qualified for training to become a firefighter had been switched to that day. Chip decided to take the civil-service examination to see if he met the requirements. He scored highest in the class. Today he travels all over the country putting out wildfires. Chip had one thing in mind, but God decided on something else.

Michelle came to the Sedona Intensive to clear away her fears about having another baby. She had had twins and one of them died at birth. Working through her concerns, she and her husband, Stephen, decided to have another child. As the due date drew closer, they started thinking about what to name the baby. One night while watching *Queen Isabella of Spain* on PBS, Stephen called out to his wife, "What do you think about the name Isabella for the baby?" Just at that moment Michelle opened a box that had the name "Isabella" printed on its side. Today Michelle and Stephen have a healthy, beautiful daughter named Isabella.

Twenty-year-old Courtney and her mother, Francie, were in their car on their way shopping when Courtney started asking her mother where she could go to help kids battling alcohol and drug addictions. Within minutes, a public-service announcement came on the radio asking for volunteers to learn how to man the phones for CONTACT, a nonprofit group set up to help kids with abuse problems. Courtney called and got involved.

And here is a coincidence that led to marriage for one of my clients. Joanna and I made a date for lunch in Dallas when I was in town to see clients. Joanna, who had been widowed little more than a year, had an appointment with me before we went to lunch. As we walked to her car, she said, "Do you mind if we go to Baby Routh's? It's a new restaurant near here. They sent me a coupon for a free lunch for two." She handed me the free-lunch card washed in pink and blues.

"Let's try it," I said.

As we were waiting to be seated, a gentleman behind us was

holding a similar free-lunch coupon. He commented to us that they must have blanketed the city with the freebie and also told us in the same breath that his lunch date had canceled at the last minute.

The host heard his comment and said, "Quite the contrary. We sent only two cards from a mailing list we got from our platinum credit card company."

"What a coincidence," Joanna gasped.

"Perhaps the gods are conspiring. Since I am alone, why don't we three have lunch together, if you don't mind," the gentleman said.

I left them around two o'clock because I had other appointments. The next time I was back in Dallas, they came to counsel with me, because they had fallen in love at first sight and were getting married in a few weeks.


## Keeping a Healthy Dose of Skepticism

Craig S. Bell, in his book, *Comprehending Coincidences: Synchronicity and Personal Transformation* says that "the investigation of coincidence is a natural choice in seeking a hidden connectedness within the forces that buffet us, for the frequently dramatic nature of coincidences not only grabs our attention, it highlights the possibility of deeper meaning in life. My approach has been to postulate tentative meanings for coincidences encountered by associates or myself, then to see if present circumstances or future developments can verify the interpretations. Over time, this allows meaningfulness to be empirically validated or refuted."

What I think Mr. Bell is saying is not to give the same gravity to all coincidences. Sometimes a book may fall from the shelf, and you should simply put it back. Someone may be dialing your number as you are calling them, but nothing of significance may come from the conversation. I daresay that more coincidences are fascinating than earth-shattering. At other times we all will have those unexplainable occurrences that have great importance to us. The fact that not all events in our life are life changing does not mean that we should ignore any for fear we may miss those that are.

Wondering when a coincidence will crop up to solve some mystery for you or lead you to a job opportunity or perhaps hitch you up with a soul mate? Keep your eyes wide open and your ear to the ground, for the next significant coincidence may be a signal that God is calling you to a golden opportunity. Believe in coincidence, but keep a healthy perspective.

# CHAPTER 11

# The Language of Synchronicity

SYNCHRONICITY: A coincidence involving a crucial time element; a meaningful interaction between two people or parallel events without appointment or a plan that seem related.

I am often asked if coincidence and synchronicity are the same thing. The strict answer is no, but the concepts are related. Both coincidence and synchronicity have to do with sequences of events that seem to be both accidental and planned. Both are characterized by the seemingly chance emergence of facts that show an uncanny relationship between people, places, things, and ideas that previously seemed unconnected. But a synchronicity always involves a crucial time element. Time is its key feature. So while every synchronicity is a coincidence, every coincidence is not a synchronicity.

In Carl Jung's book *Synchronicity: An Acausal Connecting Principle,* Jung takes hundreds of near-impenetrable pages to explain what I prefer simply to call God shots in action. The Supreme Creator is putting people together in the most fascinating but unpredictable ways. There is a divine principle of magnetism that draws us together in ways that the finite mind cannot explain. As smart as scientists and engineers seem to be, which one of our advanced doctors could possibly track the telephone wires God uses to get people, places, and things together for purposeful interaction? As it is said in Shakespeare's play *Hamlet*, "There are more things in Heaven and on Earth, Horatio, than are dreamt of in your philosophy."

## Vaneta and Kelly

Vaneta couldn't shake the urge to go to Singapore. Although she knew little of the country's people and its culture, every time she saw pictures of its botanical gardens or snapshots of the Raffles Hotel, Vaneta wanted to pack her bags and get on the next plane headed east. One day her boss called her into his office in Atlanta and said that she had been requested by the director of international business affairs to head up a task force to introduce the company's newest technology in Singapore. When she heard the location, she sat down with a thud.

"What's wrong? Don't you want the assignment?" asked her senior manager.

"Of course. I was just surprised by where they want me to go."

A short time later, after packing for the trip and arriving at the airport, Vaneta discovered her flight was canceled and she had been rebooked at another time, traveling via South Africa. Upgraded to Business Elite, she was assigned to sit next to a male passenger named Kelly. Kelly was being considered for CEO at a Fortune 500 HMO headquartered in Atlanta, but he had decided to work with children and adults dying of AIDS in South Africa.

You might be thinking that this was a scene right out of a movie in which boy meets girl, they love each other at first sight, and live happily ever after. The proverbial kismet, right? Nothing could be further from the truth. Kelly found Vaneta's perfume offensive, and she thought his appearance was more suited to third class. Vaneta and Kelly were definitely opposites who did not attract. He turned his head to the window and slept through the whole flight.

Two years later, Kelly was working to educate South Africans about sexually transmitted diseases. That's when Vaneta was sent to Cape Town for a conference on communication. She ran into Kelly in a hotel lobby. This time there were no conflicts over fragrances or appearances, for time had changed both of them. They had dinner and talked until midnight about Vaneta's dissatisfaction with Singapore.

"Why did I have such a strong urge to go there?" Vaneta asked.

"Maybe you went to Singapore to meet me on the flight over," said Kelly.

"But we hated each other at first glance," said Vaneta.

Kelly asked, "Have you changed since then?"

"A ton," said Vaneta.

Following the dinner, Vaneta and Kelly stayed in touch through letters and phone calls and occasional visits. As they peeled back the layers of prejudice and criticism that had initially separated them, they changed even more: They listened to their hearts. They eventually married and came back to the United States as directors of a poverty program in Appalachia.

How could two people meet and not "get it" from the moment they laid eyes on each other? And why would God play such a cruel joke on us poor souls, anyway?

Good questions. Vaneta and Kelly needed to meet when they did, but both had a lot of growing to do. God was not playing a joke on anybody. He was paving the way. Check with high school or college chums to see how many have reunited with an old flame twenty or thirty years later when they are better able to understand each other. I know more stories about love being rekindled at school reunions or by chance encounters. What is meant to be will never be denied. Synchronicities aren't always wrapped up in a neat package. All of life's experiences are about growing and changing and facing what we need within ourselves. From time to time, circum-stances are such that two people meet and they click immediately but rarely without some trouble areas to work through. God truly works in mysterious ways—but He does work.

## Anne and William

Anne's parents were traveling cross-country to attend a funeral when her mother, who was six months pregnant with Anne, went into labor. Through a mistake in the hospital nursery Anne and baby William were switched. The error was quickly cor-rected and after a few days in the maternity ward, Anne was taken to Indiana by her parents. William's parents brought him home to a nearby town. Both infants grew up hundreds of miles apart and never saw one another again—until fate reunited them as adults.

Anne married a surgeon named Harold, who operated in a small hospital. William also married. He and his wife were visiting that town when a car hit their six-year-old son, Adam, and he sustained head trauma. Adam was rushed to the hospital, where Anne's hus-band performed the intricate surgery that saved his life. While mak-ing small talk in the cafeteria after the surgery, Anne and William discovered their connection.

"My mother would say every time I went home to visit, 'Wonder whatever happened to baby William?' " said Anne.

"My mother used to say that she could have been raising a little red-headed girl named Anne if the hospital had not discovered their error," said William.

God spoke in this instance with actions, not words. Only through the unfathomable nature of synchronicity did William and his family hook up with Anne's husband, who had just completed advanced training in a revolutionary technique perfectly suited to treat Adam's head injury.

"I am the only board certified physician in the country at the moment who is able to do what I did with Adam," Harold told William and his wife.

What are the odds of two people reconnecting as Anne and William did? And how likely is it that Anne would be married to the only doctor certified to perform the surgery Adam needed? One million to one odds? Probably higher. But God knows no odds. He confirms his magical powers every day through extraordinary synchronicities.

## Roseanne and Rick

Roseanne and Rick met on a blind date. She was working for a cosmetics company and traveled all over the world while Rick was a troubleshooter for an insurance company based in London. She lived in New York and Minneapolis was his home, but they were introduced in Munich, Germany. Having been married and divorced before she was thirty, Roseanne was not looking for a long-term relationship but rather some tender, loving care. Ten minutes into the dinner with the couple who had set them up on the date, Rick was showing photographs of the new house he had bought when Roseanne let out a gasp.

"My God, is 333 your house number?" she said, pointing to the numbers on the door of the house in the photograph.

"Yes," answered Rick. "Anything wrong?"

"Three-three-three is *my* house number," said Roseanne.

Although Roseanne had been adamant about no serious involvement, the couple married six months later and decided to keep both No. 333 houses, since they continued to travel with their respective jobs. Roseanne clearly felt she had experienced both a synchronicity and a sign and had opened her mind to happiness.

## Nothing Is Beyond Possibility

There was absolutely no reason for these synchronicities to have happened to Vaneta, Kelly, Anne, William, Roseanne, and Rick, but they did occur and they were all cases of God speaking in His unique, divine language. Vaneta and Kelly at first seemed star-crossed, but ended up spending their lives together. Anne and William were brought together for William's son's miracle healing by Anne's husband, Harold, and Roseanne and Rick found their connection through numbers.

As we begin to assemble the parts of the new language and experience them in action, nothing is beyond possibility. For as David Linnig says in his review of Robert Hopcke's *There Are No Accidents: Synchronicity and the Stories of our Lives*, "Implicit in Jung's concept of synchronicity is the belief in the ultimate 'oneness' and interdependence of the universe." Jung laid down the first bricks for building on the idea that we are all connected. I add the notion that synchronicity is God's way of getting many of us back together. The expression, "we're speaking the same language," gives rise to the idea that God has plans beyond our comprehension and that He expresses these ideas in the new language. Synchronicity is one technique in His master plan of reunion.

Hopcke had a few good suggestions for all of us as we look for synchronicities in our own lives:

1. Expect the unexpected.
2. Be open to the meaning in what you did not want to happen.
3. Get obstinate and see what happens.
4. Wander the world randomly and be willing to listen to whatever life presents.
5. Be both determined and willing to let go.

It is not important to know the reasons why everything happens in the amazing world of synchronicity. When a synchronicity happens to you, simply feel the awe. Don't be jaded. Move with the flow of the synchronicity's energy and be ready to embrace what only God can bring into your life: the majesty and magic of our interconnectedness.

CHAPTER 12

# The Language of Signs and Wonders

**SIGNS:** God gets His message across to us through billboards, post-cards, business cards, newspaper and magazine headlines, and sky-writing. He may catch our attention through the unexpected but timely appearance of an animal, an object, or event. Drama is often the flavor of the experience. And it may carry advice or encouragement.

**WONDERS:** God uses awe and spectacle to bring attention to His omnipotence. It affirms the majesty of God's creativity and infinite power. Wonderment is open to a wide variety of manifestations.

Jane had decided to move to Los Angeles from her cottage on the beach in Florida. While the building inspector was examining the cottage for a prospective buyer, serious termite damage was uncovered.

"I knew I would have to pay for the repairs," Jane said, "but I was relieved. It was as if God was saying, 'This property is condemned. It's time to leave.'"

\* \* \*

Gail was undecided about whether or not to attend a spiritual retreat in Arizona. Praying for a sign, she discovered that her father's handkerchief, which had been firmly tied to her bedpost since his death, was now lying flat on her pillow. "I felt my father was urging me on," Gail said later. She did go and called the experience the best thing she'd ever done for herself.

Before Bob and Gloria's son died of AIDS, he told his parents that he would always be with them. In the room where he died were Indian amulets and angel talismans that had a lot of feathers attached to them. Within days of his death, Bob and Gloria began to find feathers on the sidewalk, in their house, in faraway travel spots, and even when they were speaking in their support group.

"Well, folks, my son's here," Bob would say as a feather came floating to the floor in front of him.

Are these signs? Are they wonders? Absolutely. I believe each of these stories is an example of God revealing Himself to ordinary people who have problems they need to solve or who crave simple reassurance. The first two incidents are signs, and the third is a wonder of God speaking to us.

Why didn't Jane and Gail just consult someone else for an opinion about their problems? The answer is simple. They could have—but neither was inclined to do so. Jane thought her friends might not want her to move, so they may have stacked their argument in favor of her staying. Gail knew if she asked her husband, he would have told her she was perfect as she was and didn't need to attend a spiritual retreat. The signs Jane and Gail received came from the purest source: God.

A wonder carries the same majesty. If Robert and Gloria were not in a henhouse or shaking a down pillow—which they weren't— the feathers had to come from somewhere. They believed that they came from their angel son. Can they prove it? No. Do the feathers make them feel that their son is happy and able to be with them? Yes. They told me that there is no doubt in their minds that their son drops feathers from his angel wings. Would God want it otherwise?

## Rita and Dr. Garcia

Rita was on a committee in Mexico City to select students academically eligible for college scholarships. One of the terms of renewal of the financial assistance was for the student to keep his or her grades up. Rita continued to support one student who went all the way through medical school on one of the Morris Foundation's scholarships even though his grades were not always up to standard.

Several years later Rita went to her gynecologist for a pregnancy test, but the result was negative. Her doctor was convinced she had a tumor. Months later, Rita was hospitalized to have the tumor removed. The doctor performing the surgery discovered that Rita was pregnant and in fact was carrying a healthy full-term baby. He delivered the infant.

After the cesarean procedure, Rita looked up at the attending physician from her hospital bed and saw the name Jesus Garcia on his white coat.

"Are you the same Jesus Garcia who went through college and medical school on a scholarship from the Morris Foundation?" asked Rita.

"Yes, I am," answered Dr. Garcia.

"God bless you, Jesus Garcia. If I had discontinued your scholarship I would not have my baby son today."

Many times the new language is speaking to us long before we know what He is trying to tell us. Rita had no idea why she continued to support a young man's education when his grades were not up to par. Little did she know he would one day save her baby's life.

These kinds of things happen to millions of people every day all over the world. Right now perhaps a farmer in Russia is getting a sign of hope for a better crop and maybe a Sherpa in Tibet is being drawn to the top of the mountain by its majesty. You can see and hear what God has in mind for you if you are open to His language. There is no pecking order or caste system for who can hear from God. He makes Himself available to each of us when we decide we would rather hear from Him than from ourselves or other people as fallible as we are.

Nothing is too small or insignificant to warrant God's attention. A Girl Scout on my street named India says that God sends her the sign of rain to let her know when to sell her cookies. I have taken a page from India's book and now turn lots of my problems over to God—even the small stuff.

Many of us are better at finding God in the big challenges in life. If you want to see members of a community rally around one another almost divinely and selflessly inspired, check in after an earthquake. When the Northridge earthquake hit in 1993, cooperation among neighbors and strangers in the same block was amazing. Floods in the Midwest in 1998 dampened everything but man's humanity to man. If one was in trouble, the whole block was at risk. Such care and concern one person feels for another is one of God's wonders. He is coming to our aid through the generosity of spirit of the people around us.

One of the most direct ways for possible success in getting a sign or wonder is through prayer. Sit and get quiet. Make a simple entreaty to God and then wait for the answer. If you are not given a sign immediately, keep at it. The next time the phone rings, it might be your answer. The next time you meet a stranger, he or she might be a sign of confirmation for you. And when you glimpse one of God's breathtaking wonders, behold its meaning.

# CHAPTER 13

# The Language of God-by-Proxy

**GOD-BY-PROXY:** The principle that God speaks to us through other people is the underpinning of the meaning of God-by-proxy. God uses the people in our life to get our attention and get His message and guidance across.

Now that we have looked at how the new language operates through coincidences, synchronicities, and signs and wonders, let's explore how God uses the people in our lives to get across His message and guidance. God-by-proxy, as I call this occurrence, was the most commonplace experience of the new language noted by respondents to a survey I sent out in 2001 to more than 6,000 people worldwide. As you read the stories that were sent back to me, you will be as amazed as I was at how friends and strangers often convey helpful and timely directions in answer to our prayers.

## Should I Go or Should I Stay?

Marlene moved to Hawaii hoping to find her life's purpose, but after two years she felt stalemated. Try as she might she never seemed to feel at home among the spiritual seekers who purported to have found bliss there.

"Should I go or should I stay?" Marlene was asking herself as she sat outside a healing center one day waiting for an appointment. The healing center was located across the street from a deep ravine. As Marlene sat waiting she noticed a woman about to step off into the ravine. Marlene leaped up and pulled the woman to safety.

"Thank God, you were right where you were supposed to be," said the visibly shaken woman.

Understanding the literal answer, Marlene also took the deeper message to heart. The woman had unwittingly spoken to Marlene's most urgent question. The guidance the woman conveyed felt right.

## Dream Job

While on vacation in Costa Rica, Elaine was offered a job as manager of a hotel. Moving would have meant leaving her friends, selling all her worldly goods, and starting over in a Third World country more than 5,000 miles from home. Still, the beauty and easy pace of life in Costa Rica tempted her. She was burned-out working as a nurse and was hungry for a new adventure. Every day on her walks Elaine would pray, "God, what do I do about this job offer?"

One day, Elaine noticed two young men walking toward her. As they passed, one randomly said to her, "Take a chance." Startled that a stranger would unknowingly address her concern, she felt guarded. Upon examination, she recognized the statement as God's answer to her prayer. She took the job, moved her family, and had a truly rewarding experience.

## Do What You Love and the Money Will Follow

Roger wanted to make furniture, not sell pharmaceuticals. When time permitted, he made a few tables, an armoire, and some chairs, all of which sold immediately. However, turning his hobby into a career was complicated—Roger was married with two children, and his wife was expecting another baby. Every time he talked to his minister about his personal aspiration, Roger was reminded that he had a family to support.

Flying home from an out-of-town business trip, Roger sat next to a man named Eddie, who manufactured furniture in North Carolina.

"I would love to design furniture," said Roger.

"What's stopping you?" Eddie asked.

Roger explained the drawbacks of his family situation.

"Do what you love and the money will follow," said Eddie.

They chatted a few more minutes—exchanged business cards—and Roger promised to send some photographs of his furniture.

Several weeks went by, and one day Roger got a phone call from Eddie.

"I got the snapshots of your furniture. You are talented, my friend, very talented!" Eddie said. "How would you like to design for Renaissance Interiors?"

"Gosh, Eddie, I told you on the plane that I have lots of monthly expenses," Roger said.

"Do what you love and the money will follow," Eddie repeated. "I've got a designer job open and I am offering it to you. It is a risk for both of us, but I own an empty house and I'll make it part of the package."

That night Roger and his wife dined at a Chinese restaurant. They were discussing what to do about the new job opportunity.

"God has always shown us the way in the past," Roger's wife said. "Why can't we hear Him about this?"

Opening a fortune cookie, Roger broke out in a Cheshire cat grin as he handed the fortune to his wife. He read, "Do what you love and the money will follow."

Roger is now a partner with Eddie in Renaissance Interiors.

## Never Say Never

I've known Pete for a long time. I believed him every time he said that he would never be in a serious relationship again. Pete had divorced his first wife after thirty years of marriage, bought a boat, taken up golf, and slept as late as he wanted on Sundays. He seemed to enjoy being a bachelor.

One day some visiting out-of-towners—Bill, Barbara, and Betty—invited him to play golf. Between rounds the two women talked incessantly about Betty's engagement.

"And to think that I swore I would never get married again," Betty said.

"Never say never," said Barbara.

Getting annoyed by this chatter, Pete piped up, "Can we play golf, for Pete's sake?"

That night at dinner, Betty ignored Pete's outburst and gave him the card of a friend who had been a widow for four years.

"Call her. She lives nearby. I think you two might hit it off."

Pete called and they have now been dating for more than a year.

## Don't Exclude Animals!

Since a dog is considered man's best friend—and who better to be a trusted proxy—I could not resist sharing the following story.

Bolivia was a freelance writer specializing in human-interest stories. She was at her creative wit's end with no idea where to turn for a good writing assignment. One day she returned home to find a mail-carrier bag and its contents strewn all over the kitchen floor with Benz, her Labrador retriever, chomping down on a magazine. Bolivia took *Spiritual Winds* out of Benz's mouth, sat on the floor, and read it. On the second page was a block ad that read FREELANCE WRITERS WANTED. Bolivia has been writing for them for two years.

## Talking It Over with Molly

Mary Lee decided she no longer wanted to live in Dallas.

"It's too hot in the summer, too cold in the winter, and too much Texas glitter all year round. I think I'll move to San Diego, where the weather is nice 365 days of the year and everybody is plain and laid-back," she said to her friend Molly.

"Mary Lee, I used to live in San Diego and I can tell you that the weather is not always perfect and the same kind of people who live in Dallas live in San Diego. Could your itchy feet have anything to do with turning forty next month?"

Mary Lee got real quiet and with a whimper said, "Maybe."

"Well, honey. I can tell you one thing. If you don't like Dallas, you won't like San Diego."

Mary Lee stayed in Dallas and today loves buying and selling glamorous fashions to Texas ladies.

Keep your eyes open and your ears tuned for evidence of God's will working on your behalf. Especially in a moment of indecision, when someone unexpectedly or unknowingly pierces your consciousness with a bit of advice that rings true, recognize that God is speaking by proxy. If you are discerning, miracles can happen. Don't hesitate to consult a friend or counselor you trust. A second opinion can go a long way to strengthening your resolve to move toward the life of your dreams.

# CHAPTER 14

# The Language of Dreams

**DREAMS:** A dream is a series of thoughts, images, or emotions occurring during sleep—a visionary creation of the imagination. God often speaks through these movies in our mind. They are screens for powerful messages.

When I was a small boy in Mrs. Schuler's Sunday school class, the Bible stories that fascinated me most dealt with dreams. I was particularly captivated by Jacob's stairway-to-heaven dream, told in Genesis, in which God promises to give the young Hebrew "the land beneath his feet." Later on in Genesis, when Egypt's pharaoh dreams that seven gaunt cows will eat seven fat ones, the ruler prepares for famine at the urging of Joseph, a dream interpreter. "God has revealed to Pharaoh what he is able to do," Joseph says, advising that food be set aside during bountiful times.

## The Many Ways God Speaks in Dreams

God promises and God reveals, all in the language of dreams. That was true in the Old Testament as well as throughout the ancient world. "In ancient Israel, in Judaism, in the Greek world and the ancient Near East generally, dreams were frequently regarded as vehicles of divine revelation, especially the dreams experienced by priests and kings," notes the *Oxford Companion to the Bible*. Elihu in the book of Job confirms that dreams convey God's messages, despite man's lack of appreciation:

> Why do you complain to Him that He answers none of man's words, for God does speak, now one way, now another, though man may not perceive it. In a dream, in a vision of the night, when deep sleep falls on men, as they slumber in their beds, He may speak in their ears and terrify them with warnings to turn man from wrongdoing and keep him from pride, to preserve his soul from the pit, his life from perishing by the sword.

While dreams in the ancient world were viewed as important vehicles of epiphany and prophecy in God's divine message system, our modern view has shifted. Since the beginning of the twentieth century, many psychologists and scientists have deemphasized the mystical value of dreams, placing them in the domain of the laboratory and the academy. For example, physiologists look at dreams as proven patterns of brainwaves and eye motion during sleep.

However, today the world now is turning once again to the new language, which defines dreams as part of God's mother tongue, the nonverbal way He has always spoken to us. Sometimes God's guidance comes in dreams that are premonitions—they help us know and prepare for the future. Sometimes our dreams are epiphanal—they reveal the answers to an important problem. Sometimes our dreams are omens warning us of a coming problem. And in some instances we hear angel murmurs in dreams. Below are several examples of each of these types of dreams.

## Dreams as Premonitions

*Example:* Jane dreamed that she was about to enter a large stadium. Many of her coworkers were filing in ahead of her, despite the fact that everyone inside was heaving and throwing up. "I didn't want to go," Jane said. "I knew something wasn't right. So I covered my head and ran to safety." Several weeks later there was an unexpected merger and most people in the company lost their jobs. Based on the dream, Jane knew she would be safe and quickly found new work.

*Example:* Mary Lou dreamed that she was afraid to go into the maternity ward at the hospital because the nurse on duty told her that none of the babies could walk. She was pregnant with her third child. When Mary Lou told her sister her dream, she said, "I fear that something is going to be wrong with my baby." When Quentin was born, he was clubfooted. Through her dream Mary Lou was better prepared for the reality of Quentin's handicap.

*Example:* Benson dreamed it was so dark outside that he couldn't find his way. He passed a lighted store window and saw his reflection. Above his head was a big shiny star that seemed to sit on his head like a crown. "I don't know what's going on with my life, but I have a feeling that something good is about to happen." Within two months Benson landed a starring part in an Off-Broadway play and won an award.

## Dreams as Epiphanies

*Example:* During a difficult period in my life, I dreamed that I was on a train traveling through what looked like England or Scotland. In the dream I kept asking myself, "Where am I going? When do I get off the train?" A man walking up and down the aisle periodically looked at me and said, "Stay on the train." I had been wondering about whether to move from Sedona to New York. The dream indicated that I was to stay in Sedona.

*Example:* Baxter had a dream in which he saw himself eating at a large family Thanksgiving dinner. Everyone was laughing and talking. Baxter saw three unkempt children peering in the window with hungry eyes. He got up from the table with a plate of food. He opened the window and gave the food to the children. "There are six more at home, mister," the little girl said. Baxter woke up; he was so struck by the dream that he decided to start a charity to feed the needy in his town.

*Example:* Nora dreamed that she saw her dead mother, Lila, talking about her to a group of ladies. "Nora never had time for me. My daughter is very selfish." Nora woke up and recorded her dream. She had a new conviction that she needed to work with senior citizens. Nora called Hospice and volunteered.

### Dreams as Omens

*Example:* Thad dreamed that a pickpocket tried to steal his wallet. He reacted quickly, thwarting the thief. As he walked away from the incident, he counted the money in his wallet and found that indeed the pickpocket had stolen a few dollars. "Thank heavens I still had most of my money," Thad said. A few days later he took the dream to heart when he was offered an investment opportunity that didn't feel right. He declined to invest in a certain stock that soon went bankrupt.

*Example:* Mort dreamed that he was digging for water on his newly purchased land, but all he managed to find were dry holes. He then began excavating near a flock of birds sitting on branches in a grove of trees. Mort took the birds in his dream to be an omen. "I noticed a clump of tree stumps on the edge of my property. I started to dig and found water."

*Example:* Mildred dreamed that she was driving her ten-year-old Ford in a downpour. The oil light on her dashboard started blinking, and the engine began to smoke. The car stalled on a remote road. When she woke up, Mildred understood the dream to be an omen to get a health checkup. She went to her doctor and found out she had high blood pressure. "I had not had a checkup in a long time. It was fortunate that I went to see Dr. Ford."

## Angel Murmurs in Dreams

*Example:* A client named Melanie dreamed that she distinctly heard a voice whisper, "Melanie, let go." Melanie had been debating whether to try to make her marriage work or to end it. She called her lawyer to start divorce proceedings.

*Example:* Martha needed to find some financial statements for her accountant. Look though she may, she came up empty-handed. One night she dreamed that she and her deceased husband were cleaning out boxes and throwing out clutter. She sat down in a chair and leaned her head back and a voice whispered, "Green." When she woke up she went out to the garage and in the corner under paint tarp was a file cabinet. Stenciled on it was the name Green. Martha opened the bottom drawer and found the papers she needed.

*Example:* Zack was upset over losing his job and his marriage at the same time. Unable to eat or sleep, he learned how to meditate. Gradually he was able to get a good night's sleep. As he slept, he dreamed that he was skiing in the mountains of France with friends. Although he was a seasoned skier, he kept falling. As he lay in the snow he heard a voice say, "Peace." "From the moment I woke up that voice seemed to calm me down and I stopped worrying about finding a job." Zack soon found work as a consultant.

Knowing what our dreams mean involves understanding a language that is symbolic. As Robert H. Hopcke writes in *A Guided Tour of the Collected Works of C. G. Jung,* "Dreams do not speak in the verbal or logical language of waking life, but rather find their voice in quite a different language, the language of symbolism. To understand dreams, therefore, one must learn to speak this language, the language of the unconscious, with its rich symbols and archetypal imagery."

You may be asking yourself how you deal with symbols if you don't know what they mean. The pharaoh probably asked himself this same question before calling in Joseph to explain why the gaunt cows in his dream were eating fat ones. In ancient times, when civilization was new and mankind was finding its mystical footing, intuitives such as Joseph demonstrated what a divine treasure trove a dream could be. Joseph's knack for the new language not only helped to save a kingdom but earned him a shining role in Old Testament history.

More recently, the Swiss psychologist Jung earned his own role in history by identifying the archetypal symbols in the landscape of the unconscious. While helping lay the groundwork for dream interpretation, Jung wisely realized that dreams have a "symbolic individuality that could best be interpreted by the dreamer and no one else," according to Hopcke. "Thus, Jung gave the dreamer's associations to the symbols and images paramount importance."

One book that especially edified my thinking about the dreamer's central role in dream work is *Jungian Psychology Unplugged: My Life as an Elephant* by Daryl Sharp, a graduate of the Jungian Institute in Zurich. Taking a stand against the dream experts, Sharp declares that "routine recipes and definitions such as those found in dream 'dictionaries' are of no value whatever." He suggests that the appearance of a tree or a rug or a snake or an apple in a dream has a unique significance depending on the dreamer. What clicks for the dreamer is what's right.

Hopcke's and Sharp's ideas resonate with me. While much can be learned from dream analysts and books, each of us must determine for ourselves what our dreams are saying. Dreams speak ultimately to our inner knowing. It is what the dream is saying to the dreamer—who may have the experience of insights and revelation—that is most important. Although we may choose to share our dreams with others to gather their thoughts and reactions, each of us is ultimately responsible for deciding what message we get. If the power is to pass from the few to the many, we must take charge of the divine content of our dream life. Let's not abdicate our power. In so doing, we may miss the chance to restore our sometimes weakened relationship with our Creator. My belief is that the deep stillness of sleep may allow God's angels to restore the telepathic lines that deliver His divine messages. Perhaps someday our scientists may prove that sleep is a spiritual activity where we get a divine tune-up.

## Tapping into the Meaning of Your Dream

Techniques to help us recall our dreams can be invaluable. I like some of the suggestions published by the Lucidity Institute in Palo Alto, California, which studies dreams and the benefits of remembering them. Here's what the institute says to do before sleeping:

1. Relax yourself completely—use your favorite relaxation tape or some peaceful music.
2. Establish an intention to remember your dream. Let a thought surface, such as "I will remember my dream."
3. Plan on waking up slowly and peacefully. It's ideal to wake up without an alarm clock or without someone rousing you.
4. Keep a pencil and paper by your bed so you may write down your dreams. However, a tape recorder with a voice-activated microphone is the optimal tool to record your dreams. You are less likely to censor your dreams and reactions to them when describing them verbally.

Point four begs the question of keeping a dream journal. Capturing your dreams on paper in order to revisit them to see recurring themes and symbols may help you to intuit what God is trying to say to you. Ask questions of yourself about everything you are able to recall from your dream, and record your thoughts and feelings with stream-of-consciousness writing. Make no judgment about what you put on the paper. Let it flow. Treat your dreams as you would a language that you are learning to speak. Get familiar with the Glossary of the New Language (see page 44), and be aware when you spot one or more of God's methods in your dreams. When something rings true for you, underline it. Your inner knowing is being stimulated.

It is natural to discuss dreams with friends and loved ones, whose insights can be beneficial if kept in perspective. However, I do have a few suggestions for proceeding: If you are receiving comments about your dream from someone else, remember that you are ultimately the expert on your own dream life. No authority reigns greater. If you are offering an interpretation of someone else's dream, remember always to preface your remarks with the words, "If that were my dream," before you forge ahead.

It is very freeing to think that you don't need a graduate degree in dreams and symbols and their meanings to understand your dreams but can use your own intuition and telepathy to hear what God is saying to you. If you can stop thinking that everybody knows more than you do, perhaps you can start listening to yourself and begin to trust your inner knowing.

## Daydreams

It is not uncommon for many of us to daydream. As a child, I loved to stare out the window and daydream, though it was often belittled. "Concentrate on what you're doing," my teachers used to say. There was little tolerance in society then toward letting the mind wander, and societal tolerance to daydreams is still low today.

It's time to develop a new respect for daydreaming—to follow our daydreams where they lead. Daydreaming is a bridge that can take us into a meditative state. It may even be considered a form of meditating while awake.

Daydreams may also help us manifest our deepest hopes. Since by definition daydreaming is a visionary creation of our imagination, it allows us to be free of the constraints of reality—to see ourselves in situations that heretofore we had only dreamed about. For instance, who of us has not daydreamed about winning the lottery or being able to live in our dream house or falling in love? By creating scenarios in our daydreams in which these desires manifest, we can perhaps find a way to make our heart's desire a reality. For example, Elaine, a graduate of the Sedona Intensive, daydreamed about quitting her job and going back to school to become an architect. Two weeks later she answered an ad for an architect's assistant. Within two weeks her boss offered to pay her tuition to go to night school to become an architect.

In his fictional masterpiece, *The Alchemist*, Paulo Coelho weighs in on the subject, urging self-reliance for the dreamer.

"You came so that you could learn about your dreams," the old gypsy says to the shepherd boy in the story. "And dreams are the language of God. When he speaks in our language, I can interpret what he has said. But if he speaks in the language of the soul, it is only you who can understand."

The young shepherd follows his dream to the pyramids in Egypt. Though he expects to find gold there, he comes up empty. When he asks why he had to go to the pyramids for nothing, the answer on the wind was, "If I had told you, you wouldn't have gone to the pyramids. Aren't they beautiful?"

Your dreams may take you on an adventure whose purpose is not readily revealed. In the end it's your choice whether or not you listen to the language of God and make the journey.

CHAPTER 15

# Confirming What You Hear

IN YOUR QUEST TO HEAR the messages of the new language, it is extremely important to keep your rational reasoning skills attuned. Lest you get the wrong impression from all the examples I've provided throughout the book, let me assure you that it is not my desire to convince you that every movie, newspaper story, or overheard conversation carries a message from God. In fact, the majority of what reaches our eyes and ears through popular culture definitely is not from God's lips.

How, then, can we know what messages are intended for us? Those who are new to knowing what they hear when they listen and what they see when they look need to proceed cautiously. Listen with a dose of healthy skepticism to distinguish between God's messages and psychobabble. Analyze each situation on its own merit and then check in with yourself. Ask "Is this premise sound?" "Do I get a definite yes or no when I question myself about this person or thing or idea?"

To achieve discernment, to look and hear with balance and integrity, I suggest you:

1. Pray daily. This allows you to stay in God's grace.

2. Meditate daily. This helps you to still your mind and to be clear and receptive.

3. Check in with yourself frequently. This lets you be your own point of reference.

4. Develop inner knowing. For example, monitor your ability to discern when a person or situation is right for you. This helps you to move forward with peace of mind.

5. Stay grounded. To help you do this, make a conscious effort to restrain compulsive behavior. This will prevent you from becoming a sheep who follows the crowd when the crowd goes overboard.

When I moved to Sedona in 1983, the New Age movement was just getting started. Everyday someone wanted me to come to a high noon meditation. I like to meditate alone.

At the time, a cluster of spiritual seekers in Sedona, dressed all in white, referred to themselves as walk-ins, a euphemism for new souls that took over their bodies, while the old ones walked out— usually during an illness or a deep depression. The idea that you could trade in a soul like you do a car struck me as crazy. And I was enraged when I heard that senior citizens were considered too old to be eligible for a walk-in but not too old to give money to the cause. Many seniors gave donations to these charlatans until the police moved in.

Over and over again I want to emphasize that it is what you believe, guided by sound moral principle, that is important. If all of your choices happen to agree with other people's ideas, fine. If not, don't be bullied or coerced into joining or espousing something that doesn't feel right to you. Stand your ground.

What is right for me may not be right for you. I don't want to convince anyone of anything. My goal and mission is to let the power pass from the few to the many. I want people to take back their power. I have great faith in people—sometimes more faith than they have in themselves. With time to learn from mistakes and listen to what your gut tells you, you will make better choices and learn when to listen and when to shut out people and their ideas. Know what you know to be true for you through experience.

## The Three Red Flags

When I am trying to practice discernment, the three red flags that I always watch out for are ego, money, and power. All are potentially corrupting influences that make me look inside to search my feelings. Before I act on anything, I ask, "Is this person doing what they're doing for self-promotion?" I try to look and listen independent of what's in and what's hot, to let concepts and ideas pass the test of time.

Here's an example: I picked up the Sunday edition of *The New York Times Magazine* today and read two stories. In the first piece, journalist Diane McWhorter had written about the recent trial in Birmingham of a former Ku Klux Klan member who was found guilty of murdering four black Sunday School girls in a bomb blast at the 16th Street Baptist Church in 1963. Elyton Village, where I grew up, was only ten blocks from the church. The story really touched me. I felt that God was reminding me that, although I try to be color-blind, there are still a lot of people who discriminate along the lines of race, creed, and color. "Practice tolerance and speak out for unity" is what God was saying to me.

The second story I read was called "Oprah of the Other Side." It was a profile of psychic John Edwards, who purports to talk to the dead. The article reported that the Sci Fi channel was going to launch Edwards in his own syndicated television show, *Crossing Over*. Now, I don't know whether or not John Edwards really talks to the dead. I've never met the man or seen him at work, but the jour-

nalist who observed Edwards working with a live television audience reported that he was less than 50 percent accurate in the messages he delivered. The show chose to edit out his failures. That
made me suspicious. Don't the producers want me to see his fallibil-
ity? Why not? If we knew his misses as well as his hits it would make
him more human.

I checked in with myself to see how I felt. I decided that
whether or not Edwards is real, I believe that life is eternal and that
each of us can develop our potential to communicate.

Here's a checklist of questions to help you make better choices
as you navigate your day and benefit from the new language.

1. Do you check in with yourself?
2. Did you detect ego, money, or power as motivations of
   the messsages?
3. What was your gut reaction to the message?
4. Did you feel more at peace after receiving the message?
5. Did the message ring true?

Remember, forewarned is forearmed: Be open to what you hear,
but exercise prudence and discernment. Be as aware of your gut
reaction to messages as you are to what your head is telling you.
While God is ever present, there is a lot of misinformation in our
world that you can instantly discard.

# CHAPTER 16

# Questions Worth Asking

UNDERSTANDING THE DYNAMICS of the new language can make you more aware of what God is trying to say to you about the changing landscape around you and how to connect with it. It can provide you with guidance for all issues great and small, but it also cries out for you to ask yourself a simple question that underlies much of all experience: What is your purpose in life?

God has a plan for each of us—including you. I ask you to probe deeper into the purpose of your life. These questions are an attempt to help you see what is on your mind and in your heart.

What would you do if you could do anything in the world?

What is standing in your way?

Does your dream require more education?

Is what you want to do possible?

Would what you want to do hurt anyone else?

Are you willing to sacrifice to live your dream?

If you are content with your life, what more can you do?

Is there a secret formula for achieving happiness?

## What Would You Do
## If You Could Do Anything in the World?

When I was a little boy, my third-grade teacher, Mrs. Cooper, told me something I have never forgotten: "Albert, God did not make anybody else quite like you. We are all different. And the plan God has for you, nobody can carry out quite as good as you can." I don't know whether I believed Mrs. Cooper then, but I do now. Few of us will grow up to be president of the United States or become a rock star. I'm not even sure that many of us are up to the challenge or would want to be. The unique soul you are—with all your potential to achieve—is God's gift to you. Becoming who He created you to be—whatever and whoever that is—is your gift back to God.

I want you to write on a piece of paper exactly what you want to do in life. You may be old or middle-aged or young. It is never too late or too early to make a plea to God for your heart's desire. I want you to put the paper under your pillow and sleep on the question until you get an answer. God will answer you. He is your Creator, but also your coach and encourager.

When I was first getting sober, I slept on what I had written for more than a year. My heart's desire read: "I want to be of service. God, give me the wisdom and the grace to lead by following. Make me willing to learn from those who come to me for guidance as I am led by their openness to finding the path that you have laid out for them."

The result was that God jump-started my life as a spiritual adviser to those who needed my help. I didn't know exactly what I wanted to do, but God did. And because I was willing, His plan was revealed to me through others.

## What Is Standing in Your Way?

Fear has always been the biggest deterrent to spiritual growth, and we are each responsible for our own roadblocks. I heard in recovery rooms that F-E-A-R stands for False Evidence Appearing Real. That definition sure worked for me. When I was able to remove the roadblocks and get into the magic and miracle of going where God led, faith took me where fear once shut me out.

How did I get past my fears, and more important, how can you get past yours? It may sound funny, but you need a box. It can be a shoe box, a hatbox—any kind of cardboard container, not more than twelve to fourteen inches long. Cut a six-inch straight line in the lid. Make it accessible for small pieces of paper. Cover the box and lid with wrapping paper, and mark it, "God Box."

Write a fear down on a small piece of paper, fold, and put the piece of paper into the box. Don't scrimp on fears. Put them all in the box. Leave them there. They are God's business now—not yours. If you ask God to help you dispose of them, I believe He will. You can clean the box out once a year. Read them as you do, for you will laugh at what you once feared.

## Does Your Dream Require More Education?

If you are a secretary but would rather teach kindergarten, ask those who know what you have to do to make it happen. If you need to finish college, investigate where you can get your degree, get an application, and find out when classes start. There are grants, scholarships, and student loans available that might make your dream simpler and easier to obtain.

If you have spent twenty years as an accountant but would rather raise horses in Texas, go after it with good, orderly planning. You may need to learn the ropes from a rancher, but you can do anything if you are acting on what God wants you to do.

Your need for more education may take a few days, not a four-year degree. There are weekend or weeklong seminars to teach you how to enhance your personal and professional life. For example, here in Sedona a psychotherapist with a background in finance conducts seminars on how to create a rosier economic bottom line by bolstering your self-esteem. Many skilled practitioners offer two-day workshops with insights into making relationships with your family or business associates more effective. And the most fascinating thing about these sessions is that many of their instructors put God in the middle of the process.

## Is What You Want to Do Possible?

Robert Browning's encouraging words, "Oh that a man's reach should exceed his grasp, or what's a Heaven for?" come to mind when I considered this question. Breaking through restraining walls in many fields of endeavor is possible, but you do not want to set impossible goals that may frustrate you. I say at times that I would like to quarterback the Dallas Cowboys, but I'm sixty-four and the coach would laugh me out of the stadium. A good friend of mine says that she wishes she could dance with the American Ballet Theatre. At forty-seven her body can't accommodate her. My point is that many things are out of reach. Age is only one factor. But if you want to do something creative or to be of service, there are no limits.

Can you paint or write as an avocation? Absolutely. Will you be able to make a living at either one? To answer that question, you would need to seek out a professional opinion and have your talent evaluated before you make the leap. For example, going from the corporate structure to self-employment can be risky but worth it if you've evaluated what you want to do, determined that you can fare well in the field, and decided where you want to start a business. In short, do your homework. Sit down and analyze your finances and your debt load and come to a rational conclusion.

All good plans are well thought out and meticulously executed. Eva, a fifty-three-year-old friend of mine in Sedona, applied to teach in China. She has been delayed, but the government agency assures her that she has a position in one of the provinces. No matter what they are telling her, she is not going to fly to China hoping she'll have a job when she gets there. She has a valid passport and a visa, and has taken all her shots, but she's staying home until she gets a confirmation of a position.

## Would What You Want to Do Hurt Anyone Else?

If you are single and your dream is to quit your job, sell your house, and move halfway around the world to plant and harvest organic vegetables, no one is stopping you. But if you are married, buried in bills, and overmortgaged you may want to pay down your debts and then talk to your family to see if your desires coincide with theirs. When there is no one to consider but you, you are more mobile and carefree. But a family should make such a decision together with a collective sense of responsibility and sacrifice. For example, from time to time, parents are willing to uproot and move across the country to New York for their daughter to study at Juilliard or their son to train in Colorado Springs with an Olympic gymnastics coach. Being willing to see who and for what God is calling is the payoff for learning to hear when you listen.

## Are You Willing to Sacrifice to Live Your Dream?

All recommendations for going where God is leading have an element of risk. To be able to weather the doubts and fears, you must have faith that God has a plan for your life and be willing to do your part to get there.

Getting out of what may be a dead-end situation requires that you know what sacrifices you might have to make. Going back to school after having had a well-paying career in advertising will require a new budget and giving up a lot of extras. You may have to adjust to cafeteria food after having acquired a taste for fine dining.

Your wardrobe may have to last you until you get that degree, and vacations may consist of picnics in the local park rather than the sunny beaches of Maui. Doing what you've always wanted to do but lacked the faith and wherewithal is worth the sacrifices you'll have to make. You may be about to discover that the best things in life really are free.

## If You Are Content with Your Life, What More Can You Do?

Not everyone wants or needs to make drastic changes in his life. If you are content, perhaps the things that are important in your life are working very well. Many who seek a spiritual life find that things fall into place for them in an orderly fashion. They accept life and take their good fortune in stride. If you are a person like this, take heart. Being satisfied with your lot—home, career, marriage, and other relationships in your life—signifies that you found God's will early on. God reminds me all the time, "I don't care where you work or where you live. I care *how* you work and *how* you live."

Learning to speak the new language is not about waiting for a call as much as it is about receiving daily suggestions to make your life better. Someone once told me that so many of us can climb mountains, ford streams, dig our way out from an avalanche of debt, rehabilitate ourselves from a critical illness, and conquer any number of impossible situations. But let someone look at us wrong, pull out in front of us in traffic, or erode our self-confidence with a thoughtless word, and we go to pieces. Checking in with God for tips to avoid folderol of all kinds makes sense. The new language is about developing a deeper awareness about everything.

## Is There a Secret Formula for Achieving Happiness?

When I hear a question like this one, I am reminded of explorer Ponce de León's search for the fountain of youth or medicine's quest for a cure for cancer. The former was sheer folly and the latter may just be a matter of science currently looking in all the wrong places. Could the answer to where to find happiness have been born within us? Is it possible that eternal youth is a state of mind? Did God bury within us antidotes for what ails us—hopeful we will go on a quest to look for what is lost? The answers to these questions can be found by silencing the noisemakers that have deafened the new language.

You must come to your own awakening in your own time. I learned this years ago when I was at a sobriety meeting with several other newcomers. A navy lieutenant, who I thought was taking alcoholism a bit too lightly, was speaking. He was laughing throughout his talk—he found humor in everything. Being a more serious fellow, I felt the lieutenant was being silly. "This man does not seem to get how dire this disease is," I said to myself.

After he was through talking, I went up to him and told him exactly how I felt about his talk.

"Albert Einstein tied his shoelaces a different way every day. I have one suggestion for you, dear fellow. The next time I run into you, make me laugh."

That was the best advice I ever got in recovery. Not taking others or myself too seriously healed me more than anything else did.

If you want to know where happiness lives, recognize that it is within you. If you want to know how to swim in its healing waters, remove the negatives in your life. The next time you get frustrated when looking for a message in all the places I have suggested, see the humor in everything and have a good laugh.

CHAPTER 17

# What It Means to Pray

SONDRA GREW UP IN LOS ANGELES, where she attended Sacred
Heart Catholic Church and graduated from Saint Xavier High
School. She said the Hail Mary every day, memorized hundreds of
prayers, and was steeped in liturgy and the rules of catechism. Yet
when her three-year-old child fell into the swimming pool and
nearly drowned, she cradled him in her arms and called out, "God,
please help me. Please save Jason." As Sondra prayed, she rocked
Jason back and forth, patting the child's back. Within minutes Jason
began to cough, spitting up water as he cried, "Mommy, Mommy."

Leigh had been out of work for three months. To try to find
some answers to his dilemma, he would take long walks in the
woods and let his mind roam in an undirected stream of consciousness. "On one channel in my head," he once explained, "I would
hear myself ask, 'What can I do about this?' My worries would float
up to the surface, and I would remember that the economy is bad
and unemployment is up. On another channel I sometimes got messages like, 'Everything's going to work out. Have faith. Go forward.'
That encouragement pushed me to send out those résumés on my
desk."

Though Sondra and Leigh were using different approaches, both were praying. Sondra talked to God in her own words about her own needs rather than following rote ritual to get God's attention. Leigh had learned to tune in to the conversations taking place in his head, trusting himself to distinguish between God's messages and the freewheeling ideas born of his own mind and our fear-based culture.

In our modern world, the definition of prayer depends on who you ask. According to the *American Heritage Dictionary of the English Language*, prayer is "a reverent petition made to God." Larry Dossey, MD, former chief of staff of Humana Medical City Dallas, writes in his book *Healing Words: The Power of Prayer and the Practice of Medicine* that "the two commonest forms of prayer are *petition*, asking something for one's self, and *intercession*, asking something for others." Dossey also defines "prayers of *confession*, the repentance of wrongdoing and the asking of forgiveness; *lamentation*, crying in distress and asking for vindication; *adoration*, giving honor and praise; *invocation*, summoning the presence of the Almighty; and *thanksgiving*, offering gratitude."

Theologian Ann Ulanov and Professor Barry Ulanov state in their book *Primary Speech: A Psychology of Prayer* that prayer is the most fundamental and important language humans speak. "Prayer starts without words and often ends without them. Prayer works some of the time in signs and symbols, lurches when it must, leaps when it can, has several kinds of logic at its disposal."

If you are anything like me, hearing that there's more than one way to pray is reassuring. Memorized prayers often instill in me a sense of duty rather than sincerity. My best times with God are when I pray in the most direct language I know. In addition, when I approach God with the innocence of a child, my willingness to listen is greater.

Beyond the dictionary's definition of prayer, or even Larry Dossey's or Ann and Barry Ulanov's, I have come to accept an even more expansive definition of prayer. I invite you to consider that thinking and praying are the same thing—both are pulses of energy forming power lines that carry our intentions to God and out into the universe. Getting quiet in meditation may steady my mind and setting a time to pray may strengthen my habit of trying to speak to God in a very deliberate fashion, but in the largest sense of its meaning, prayer has no beginning and no end. Anytime I am thinking, I am also praying. As my thoughts convey my emotions, desires, and intentions, that constitutes prayer.

Prayer is not just a classical form of entreaty. In many Western religions, God is considered an outside force to whom we send our prayers, and He may or may not act upon our entreaty. I find this concept of God and prayer demeaning to human nature. Prayer is all of what we think. Our thoughts, feelings, aspirations, dreams, and intentions—whether deliberate or unintentional—belong in the category of prayer.

As I have likened prayer to energy running across power lines, I believe each of us exists in a kind of electrical force field that is created by our thoughts. If our thoughts emerge from bloated egos, narcissism, negative drives, and emotions, we create static and interference that can block our reception of God's voice. To keep the telepathic power lines to God in good repair, we need to keep our thoughts constructive and positive. In chapter six, we worked on clearing away the old static that had accumulated in our childhoods. As we go forward, prayer can be the way we stay in alignment with who we really are and what God has created us to do.

When you begin to pray and meditate, it is beneficial to have a few familiar prayers and to set aside time every day to practice stilling the mind. Steady routines are useful for beginners. But practicing thinking and praying is much like taking the training wheels off a bicycle when you learn to ride. The longer you pray, the sooner you can depart from the regimen of instruction and do what works for you. From my experience with clients, more people want to use their own method and need to be free of the rigidity of the church, temple, or mosque of their childhood.

## Encouraging Prayer as Every Thought

Following is a list identifying several types of prayers to help you get started.

1. There are prayers of *petition:* asking something for one's self. Jolene prayed for a job that would help support her children and herself. Some called her prayers selfish, but she knew that she must entreat the true source of every-thing, God.

2. There are prayers of *intercession:* asking something for others. The World Council of Churches prayed for peace on earth and religious tolerance. Whereas man had been unsuccessful in making peace, God could bring nations together—He could intercede on mankind's behalf.

3. There are prayers of *confession.* Mark prayed he had phys-ically harmed his children and been unfaithful to his wife. His admission in a prayer of confession made it pos-sible for him to get counseling so that he could change his behavior.

4. There are prayers of *lamentation.* Simon regretted his thoughtless acts of unkindness. The more he prayed the less he acted cruelly to others. His prayer of lamentation was a reminder that God could soften his heart and open him to change.

5. There are prayers of *adoration.* Ansel prayed for the abil-ity to deepen his love of God. The more he felt the rap-ture of that relationship, the stronger was his resolve to do God's will.

6. There are prayers of *invocation*. Allyson prayed daily, "God grant me the serenity to accept the things I cannot change, courage to change the things I can, and the wisdom to know the difference." She invoked God's peace in her life.

7. There are prayers of *thanksgiving*. John's daily prayer at the dinner table was, "God, bless this food to the nourishment of our bodies and our bodies to those they service. We thank you for all you provide. Amen."

From the time that prayer and meditation became a daily habit for me, I have come to realize that prayer is a running commentary directed to God and my fellow man, and includes every single thing about which I am concerned. The dialogue is often silent and takes place in my head. Other times I talk out loud. It doesn't matter. God can hear me just as well in the thunder of silence as when I make loud pronouncements in a group setting. What I have gotten away from is the need to impress God with techniques of invocation. I agree with the man who said that the most powerful prayer he ever prayed was, "God, help me!"

As you become more aware that all consciousness is prayer, pay attention to all the thoughts in your head. What does your thought process consist of? Is it full of optimism, joy, and positive expectations or do your thoughts reflect pessimism, worry, dread, jealousy, and resentment? Do you wish harm or seek revenge on others in your head? If so, then I believe you are praying to harm someone. Vindictive thoughts are prayers of ill intention. They are impulses of energy that surround us with static—worse, they can cause damage.

Wise men have suggested that the only prayer that really works is, "Thy will, not mine, be done." Such a prayer acknowledges that God knows best how to reconcile everything. Yet always safeguard your thought process. Evict the negative, hurtful thoughts, and keep your thought stream as upbeat as possible. Don't forget to ask for God's help.

It is the momentum of prayer and its continuum in your daily life that empties you of selfishness and unwillingness to listen when God speaks. Keep nurturing yourself with prayers as you look for God's direction in your life.

# CHAPTER 18

# Thy Will Be Done

WHEN JOCELYN'S EIGHTEEN-YEAR-OLD SON, Gary, slipped into a coma following a car wreck, she organized several prayer vigils all over the city. A local radio deejay picked up on Gary's plight, and the petitions to God for his recovery skyrocketed. Even kids got into the act, washing cars to raise money to defray his medical expenses. Every person touched by Gary's story seemed to be joined in asking God to let Gary live. But after three weeks of heroic struggle, Gary died.

As my mother Maggie lay dying in intensive care in Saint Vincent's Hospital at the age of eighty, I held her hand, kissed her cheeks, and brushed her snow-white hair. Though Mother had had a stroke and could not speak, I talked with her about many of the humorous incidents that had happened throughout our shared lives and even sang songs she loved. In my private moments, I asked God with great fervor to spare my mother's life, to let us have more time together. But at three o'clock one Saturday morning in March, I felt mother's spirit leave her body.

The desire to hold on to our loved one as long as we can is universal. Everyone has a story of a life taken too soon. But oftentimes death is the kinder route an illness can take. Had my mother lived, the doctors said it was unlikely she would ever have regained consciousness. Knowing Mother and her cherished sense of dignity, such a compromised survival would not have been her choice.

It is human nature to pray that someone lives through an illness or survives an accident. We want to hear those magic words, "We got it all," or "He's going to make it." Who wants to deal with the worse-case scenarios that life serves up? Who wants to leave it in the hands of God if the outcome can be tilted with an avalanche of prayers? In the case of Gary, he was only eighteen. His whole life was ahead of him. Being unattached to the outcome of Gary's accident—whether he lived or died—was unthinkable and unnatural for his family and friends. When my mother died, her death was easier to accept because she was eighty. But I still prayed for her to live.

## Prayerfulness

Larry Dossey, in discussing prayer in his book *Healing Words*, says that some of us "live with a deeply interiorized sense of the sacred, which could be called a spirit of *prayerfulness*, a sense of simply being attuned or aligned with something higher." Prayerfulness is "accepting without being passive, is grateful without giving up. It is more willing to stand in the mystery, to tolerate ambiguity and the unknown. It honors the rightness of whatever happens, even cancer." Dossey feels that many of us are trying to "tell God what to do" in our prayers of intercession, at such time as when we ask God to let Gary live, to spare Maggie a little while longer.

In my own prayer life, I have come gradually to use the words, "Thy will be done." It's my signal to God that He knows better than I do. I am not suggesting that you should not pray your way, or for a specific outcome, if that is the route you feel is most natural. Everything in life is a process, not a formula. Nor am I saying that you should pray in lieu of taking reasonable actions that may remedy your situation, especially proven medical steps. Remember that

Larry Dossey talks about "accepting *without being passive* [italics added]." I agree. I do not advocate a fatalistic dependence on prayers alone.

Though we pray and seek God's guidance, the action we take or the action we decline is our choice to make. Each of us governs our own life. To govern is to choose. Free will has the accompanying obligation of personal responsibility. There will undoubtedly be times when we are called upon to exercise the right use of will to resolve an emergency or crisis. We may pray to God for guidance in those situations, but the responsibility to choose to act or not is ours and ours alone.

For instance, I recently read of a man in California who had been in a coma for more than ten years, unable to see, hear, speak, or feed himself—he was comatose with no hope of ever living without twenty-four-hour care. His wife chose to take him off life support, and a judge sanctioned her decision. She did not wait for him to die a natural death; rather, she chose to free him from the shackles of a living death. In cases like these, using one's own free will seems to be appropriate.

## Living Life on Life's Terms

There are times when praying for a specific outcome—and getting it—may prove more difficult in the long run. Let's return for a minute to Gary.

If Gary's family and friends had known that he would have ended up living in a permanent coma if he survived, do you think they might have prayed, "Thy will, not mine, be done?" To pray for God's will also prepares you to pray for help to bear whatever will follow.

Floating around these days is a mistaken concept that illnesses or accidents imply spiritual shortcomings. The way this thinking goes, you got sick because you were somehow not whole or fit enough or good enough. Nothing could be further from the truth. So let us agree, if someone dies, they have not been punished. Perhaps to live would have been a punishment. Or perhaps the sacrifice of their life has a higher purpose.

For example, Angela was a three-year-old girl who vanished without a trace from her backyard in Miami. Although her parents tried everything—including prayer—to try to find their daughter, the child has not been found after three years of searching. Although everyone prayed for her safe return, those prayers went unanswered. How did Angela's mother handle her grief? She started a program to build greater awareness among minority mothers and caregivers of the importance of always knowing where their children are, and a hotline to help look for missing infants. Perhaps with Angela's disappearance, the lives of thousands of other children have been saved.

Another example is John Walsh, producer and host of Fox TV's *America's Most Wanted*. He was the father of a six-year-old son who was kidnapped and murdered. The way Walsh coped with the loss of his son was to create a television venue to publicize pictures and stories of criminals who needed to be brought to justice. In interviews, Walsh says how much he still misses his son but that he worked through his grief by helping parents who have missing and murdered children see their killers brought to justice.

Many people have discovered service in the face of tragedy and death. It is not only a means of coping, but also a chance for something positive to come out of a very tragic circumstance. I am not suggesting that anything can make up for the death of a child or anyone else, for that matter, but pain and suffering often usher in new life and tremendous possibilities. Creating an organization or venue to help others in a similar situation can be a powerful antidote for grief, sorrow, and loss.

No one knows why things happen the way they do. There is no wise man or prophet who understands what God's purpose is at the moment of any crisis, but after time goes by, someone like John Walsh finds a way to benefit society at large from his own personal tragedy.

To be able to live life on life's terms can help us find acceptance in the deepest registers of our soul in the face of the most gruesome happenstances in our lives. Trying to figure out why something happened or to pray for God to give us what we want may be to block God's infinite plan. As hard as it may be, there is great benefit in letting things be revealed. We have discussed powerlessness in chapter three and confronted ego as well in chapter four. If we are truly in the will of God, we must accept what He gives and what He takes away from us when we have no control over the matter. I am a firm believer that He does not give us more than we can handle.

While I was writing this chapter, a friend of mine named Bob, an ex-Catholic priest from Las Vegas who married a woman named Sarah ten years ago, called. He said that Sarah had what looked like terminal colon cancer and had part of her liver removed. The oncologist told Bob that she would die in a matter of weeks. But God had other plans. Praying constantly, their friends petitioned their higher power to heal Sarah, if it be God's will. Bob said that in a matter of days Sarah began first to feel heat and then the pain would suddenly stop. Not only is she in remission, but she is convinced that she has been healed through the power of prayer.

Not all prayers of petition are about life-threatening circumstances or death. Sometimes people pray for something as simple as a new house or job security. Agnes prayed that her brother Jack would not be laid off in a downsizing at his company. Her prayers did not turn the tide for her brother, as he was dismissed from his job without severance. Did he roll over and play victim? Did he blame God for Agnes's failed prayer? No is the answer to both questions. He rolled up his sleeves and started his own company. This happened seven years ago. Today he is a wealthy man working at something he loves. Agnes prayed for something specific for Jack, but God had something else in mind.

If you will turn your concerns over to God and pray your steps are guided, I believe your life will go exactly as God planned. Guide the outcome without inviting God into the process, and you may rue the day you played God.

I now begin and end each prayer with, "Thy will, not mine, be done." And whatever happens, I know that I have asked for God's will to be done in all my affairs, no matter what steps I take or decisions I make.

Let us review how we can get the most out of our prayers of petition in time of illness or death.

1. When tragedy strikes, ask God to help you bear the burden of pain or loss.

2. If possible, let go of expectations and outcomes when asking for God's help; simply pray for wisdom and guidance and that the will of God be done.

3. Look for the silver lining in everything, especially with tragedy and death.

4. Ask God to do what is best and not what you or others want, wherever possible.

5. Ask for the miracle to occur, only if this is God's will.

# Improving Your Reception
# of the New Language

IN PART I, I have shared the story of my transformation. In part II, I defined and explored the new language. Now it's your turn. In part III, I provide exercises and tools to help you clear away the interference and static that keep you from being the person you were meant to be. This process, which serves as the foundation of the Sedona Intensive, has five stages:

Stage One: Meditation—Stilling the Mind

    1. Techniques and exercises

Stage Two: Deflating Your Ego

    1. Exposing addictions and compulsive behavior

    2. Insights and exercises

Stage Three: Exposing Family Patterns

    1. An explanation of secrecy, favoritism, narcissism, rejection, and manipulation by adults, including physical harm, sexual abuse, and abandonment

    2. Insights and exercises

Stage Four: Remembering Who You Really Are

1. Becoming authentic

2. Dealing with parental projections

3. Healing the defended self

4. Reclaiming lost or buried parts of yourself

Stage Five: Practicing Forgiveness

1. Dealing with anger and rage

2. Identifying and transforming of dark emotions

3. Understanding the power of now

4. Writing forgiveness letters

# CHAPTER 19

# Now It's Your Turn
# To Still the Mind and Meditate

MANY OF US DO NOT HAVE a clear understanding of exactly what meditation is. Simply put, meditation is the focusing of one's mind in order to enhance one's ability to reflect on or ponder something. Meditation enhances our ability to view a concept or situation with continued attention. In order to do this effectively, it is helpful first to learn to still the mind.

## Meditation Preparation

### Phase I

Most people need to learn techniques to still the mind. Rather than force yourself to meditate without any preparation, I suggest that you sit quietly in the dark for a few minutes each day for about a week to get calm. Sit erect in a chair with your feet on the ground. If you like, enhance the mood by wearing an eye mask that blocks out the light. Another way to create a premeditative atmosphere is to play soft music while sitting.

When you first try to still the mind, you may feel restless and your mind will probably wander. Do not press yourself. There is no timetable for success. It takes longer for some people to relax. The mind is accustomed to busyness and distractions; Zen Buddhism refers to this frenetic mental activity as monkey mind.

There are two approaches I suggest to beginners who are trying to still the mind. You can use your mind's eye to imagine a white light, or you may want to burn a white candle. If you choose your mind's eye, envision a white light. It can be a candle flame or a shapeless, colorless light. If you burn a white candle, stare at the candle until your eyelids begin to close. This exercise helps you to still the mind and to focus on one thing. It stops random thoughts from entering your mind and allowing the mind to roam.

If you become fidgety, stop the exercise. However, note any progress you've made by sitting in the dark. Did you feel more relaxed? Was there a noticeable change in your stress level? If so, you have made a good beginning in preparing for meditation.

If possible, do this exercise at the same time every day. The more you sit quietly in the dark, the sooner your mind will cease chattering and allow the process to work.

In the beginning, if you like, do no more than sit and listen to music while looking at a glowing candle. You will know when to move on to the next phase of learning to meditate.

One suggestion for measuring the change in levels of relaxation is to keep a log of the length of time you are able to sit quietly, the time of day, and the musical selection played, as well as your thoughts on the process. Include in your journal how you feel after you are finished with each sitting. For example, you might note that you are more capable of handling difficult conversations with greater ease. The reflective aspect of quieting your mind helps you to think before you speak when communicating with others.

Some students stay in this first phase for months. Don't be impatient. You are learning, and the journey may be long but it will be rewarding.

Here is a review of checkpoints for the first phase of meditation preparation.

1. Pick a dark, quiet place.
2. Wear a mask to block out the light (optional).
3. Sit erect in a chair with feet on the floor.
4. Play soft music.
5. Focus on a white light or stare at a glowing candle.
6. If fidgety, stop the exercise.
7. Keep a log of your time spent in the exercise and how you felt.
8. Try to sit at the same time each day.

### Phase II

The second phase of preparing to meditate is abdominal breathing. You will develop a rhythm for your breathing in the following exercise, as well as an increased awareness of breath. Before beginning, please wear loose clothing and unfasten your belt or anything restrictive around your waist. You do not want to impede the breath. Also, remove your shoes.

In a darkened room, sit erect in a chair with your feet on the floor. Close your eyes. Sit as tall as possible.

Take a deep breath in through the nose . . . and hold it . . . gently exhale through the mouth. Breathe as you ordinarily do for a few seconds. Then . . . take a deeper breath in through the nose . . . and hold it a little longer . . . exhale through the mouth. With each exhalation notice the movement of your chest and be aware of your breathing pattern.

Breathe in gently through the nose . . . hold it . . . let the breath out gently. Breathe in . . . exhale through the mouth. Your eyelids will grow heavy and your jaw will go slack. Continue to breathe. Letting go . . . just relax.

Breathing deeply from the solar plexus enhances the positive flow of energy throughout the body. Shallow breathing inhibits this process. To monitor the depth of breath, place your hand gently over your abdomen to feel the breath expand and contract in this region.

Practicing breathing exercises will be a giant step toward meditation. Consistency and routine will lead to greater success as you continue learning. Practice at the same time daily, and don't forget to keep a journal.

Remember to stop the breathing exercise if you become restless. You do not want to tax yourself or force yourself to breathe beyond your limits. Forcing will cause you to give up the process.

Some beginners fall asleep. To avert this, plan to do your breathing when you are rested. Be persistent in developing good breathing habits.

This is a review of checkpoints for the second phase of meditation preparation.

1. Pick a dark, quiet place.
2. Sit erect in a chair with feet on the floor.
3. Wear loose clothing.
4. Remove your shoes.
5. Make sure you are relaxed before you begin the breathing exercise.
6. Develop a smooth, easy rhythm to your breath.
7. Place your hands gently over your abdomen to feel the breath expand and contract.

8. If you nod off, wake up and stop the exercise.

9. Do breathing exercises daily and at the same time.

10. Keep a journal of your observations and progress.

## Meditation

After consistent practice of the two preparatory exercises, you will be ready for meditation. Prepare yourself by stilling your mind in a dark, quiet place and practicing abdominal breathing. When you feel that your mind is still and you are ready to go into the meditative state, use the following brief meditation exercise for several days or weeks to acclimate yourself to the process. You may want to record the words and play them on a Walkman. Or you may choose to say your own words silently in your head. The purpose of the words, whether on a tape or spoken silently, is to guide the mind to shut out all distractions and to focus on one thought.

I am going to share with you my favorite short meditation, but you may use whatever coincides with your spiritual tradition. It may be a simple, "God, hear my prayer." Then you might go on to quote a favorite poem or passage that has inspired you. Remember that the purpose of this exercise is to help you still the mind, to contemplate a single idea, and eventually to hear God when He speaks to you. The exercise can last as little as three minutes.

### Short Meditation for Healing

*We ask the Infinite Intelligence God to put the White Light of Protection around us. Allow only the Highest and Best to come to us. For we ask in the Name of our Father who art in Heaven; hallowed be thy name. Thy kingdom come, thy will be done, on earth as it is in heaven. Give us this day our daily bread, and forgive us our debts as we forgive our debtors. And lead us not into temptation but deliver us from evil. For thine is the kingdom and the power and the glory forever. Amen.*

Remain seated with your eyes closed when you choose to end your meditation. If you are using a tape, sit until the meditation ends. Keep your mind clear.

*Now I am going to bring you out of meditation. You should feel relaxed and rested. When I count three you will open your eyes and be wide awake and alert. One. Two. Three. Wide awake. Come all the way back.*

The value of meditation is its carryover as you go about your day's work. Meditation is a clearing exercise that allows you to function better in all areas of your life. Remember, it is not the length of time you meditate that's important, it is the level of relaxation and quality of the meditation that count.

Once you become comfortable with the three-minute meditation, you may want to graduate to ten minutes. Because of the lengthening of the meditation, I suggest you tape the above meditation words three times successively and play it on a Walkman while you are sitting quietly, or use a preexisting meditation tape. Caution: Never use meditation tapes while driving. Play them only in the comfort of your home or office.

Following is a meditation I wrote and have been using in the Sedona Intensive for many years. If you like it, record it and play it for yourself. Continue to do your abdominal breathing.

### Nondenominational Ten-Minute Meditation for Healing

*Your toes are relaxed and healed. Your ankles are relaxed and healed. Your shins are relaxed and healed. And you are feeling so relaxed and so healed. Your knees are relaxed and healed. Your thighs are relaxed and healed. Your buttocks are relaxed and healed. From your waist down you are feeling so relaxed and so healed. Letting go. Be in this moment.*

*Your internal organs are relaxed and healed. Your sternum is relaxed and healed. Your spine is relaxed and healed. Feeling so relaxed. Getting a bit drowsy. You will not go to sleep . . . merely let go of all outside sounds. Your heart is relaxed and healed. Your back is relaxed and healed. Your hands and arms are relaxed and healed. From the neck down, you are feeling so relaxed, so healed and your body begins to tingle . . . feeling weightless . . . letting go.*

*Your throat is relaxed and healed. Your mouth is relaxed and healed. Your ears are relaxed and healed. Your eyes are relaxed and healed. Your entire body is feeling so relaxed, so healed. Your body is feeling weightless and a tingling sensation covers your body. Letting go. Just relax.*

*A powerful white light comes in through the top of your head, flooding the cavity of your face, moving through the chest down through your waist, down your hips. Moving down the legs, the while light emits from your right toe and a powerful neon cord of light begins to encase your entire body.*

*Outside in, inside out, your body is so relaxed, so healed, and nothing can harm you. You are in a powerful cocoon of protection. Just relax.*

*Your body begins to float, as if you were in a giant balloon. A light breeze begins to lift you up through the ceiling; you float and drift higher and higher into the sky. Looking down, you see the houses and trees and cars and people getting smaller and smaller. See how inconsequential all those people, places, and things you were worried about are? Let go of everything and everybody. Lifting and floating higher and higher into God's universe, free and safe and healed.*

*Soon you choose a cloud and will yourself to sink into it, as if*

*you were sitting on a sofa or chair. Ah . . . so soft and relaxed.*
*Just relax. Continue to breathe. Letting go.*

*Soon it begins to rain gently. The light drizzle washes away all*
*dross of the afterbirth of your healing, leaving you clear and cen-*
*tered.*

*Suddenly the rain stops and a rainbow streaks through the sky.*
*And a booming voice says, "Without the rain, there can be no*
*rainbow. Without stress and confusion, there would be no reason*
*to turn to God as your healer. God is your source and God has a*
*plan for your life. Listen each day, for His voice will speak to you*
*and lead you where He would have you go."*

Sit quietly for approximately five minutes.

*We ask the Infinite Intelligence to keep the White Light of*
*Protection around us. Allow only the highest and best to come to*
*us. For we ask this in the name of truth, love, and beauty, for*
*peace, balance, and harmony. Amen.*

*Now it is time to come back from the meditation. We ask the*
*Infinite Intelligence to keep the White Light of Protection around*
*us, continue to remove all negative vibrations and allow only the*
*highest to come to us. For we ask in the name of truth, love, and*
*beauty, for peace, balance, and harmony.*

*Silently count one, two, three. Open your eyes. Wide awake.*
*Come all the way back.*

Do not jump up immediately after your meditation. You have
been in an altered state. Allow the mind and body to slowly come
back to alert consciousness. Take five minutes to sit quietly.

Meditation can restore you emotionally, mentally, and physically. Your reaction to what people say, what you experience, and
the trying circumstances in your life will change dramatically for the
better.

The ultimate purpose of daily meditation is to reconnect to
God, to hear His voice, and follow His directions. After a year of

meditating, I noticed a big difference in my relationship to God. My prayers of petition changed drastically. My prayers began to become more of a personal talk with God, and meditation began to become listening for what He would have me do with my life. I did not have expectations in my communication with God. I prayed for God's will to be done in my life in all of my affairs. Soon I came to accept His will as whatever appeared in my life. This was truly life on life's terms, which was brand-new for me.

Although I caution clients to say simply to God, "Thy will, not mine, be done," some pray for what appear to be mundane things. I have one client who prays for her garden to flourish every spring so it can bless the lives of those who stop to smell the roses. I do not fault her. This draws her closer to God. Her method works for her.

As a child I prayed, "Now I lay me down to sleep, I pray the Lord my soul to keep. If I should die before I wake, I pray the Lord my soul to take. God bless Momma and Daddy and brothers and sisters and all the starving people of the world. Good night, God. Albert."

Whatever prayer is prayed with unselfishness and sincerity, I believe that God hears it. As it says in the Old Testament, "Man looketh on the outward appearance, but God looketh on the heart."

## Highlights of Meditation

1. Sit in a dark, quiet place with loose-fitting clothing. Remove your shoes.

2. Practice abdominal breathing before meditating.

3. If you tape the meditation, never use it while driving an automobile.

4. Start the meditation practice for three minutes until meditating becomes natural and easy for you.

Gradually build your meditation from three to ten minutes.

5. Change prayers and techniques to suit you.

6. Sit quietly for five minutes when the meditation ends.

7. To enhance the maximum benefits from meditation, meditate daily and at the same time each day.

## Meditating with Others

Once you become relaxed and you can meditate without distractions, you may choose to meditate with friends or family members. But in the beginning it is best for you to meditate alone.

Group meditation allows a healing place to clear away blocks to communication. Before going into meditation, a moderator can pick a topic for meditation. It is a tradition in the Sedona Intensive for clients to go home and organize family meditation, just as families have a set time to discuss schedules and problems.

The Daltons are a family of seven, with children ranging in age from five to seventeen. The father and mother decided to begin family discussions by sitting quietly for five minutes. Soon their high school sophomore son suggested they play music. Next they added a guided meditation. Two years later the Daltons have less confusion and arguments at family gatherings because they first clear away the static.

CHAPTER 20

# Deflating Ego

BEN IS A THIRTY-TWO-YEAR-OLD ATTORNEY who graduated with honors from Harvard and is married with two children. He coaches his son's soccer team, serves as president of the local PTA, and has been honored as citizen of the year in his small Midwest town. He is a model citizen—except when he beats his wife. He does this while experiencing dark mood swings.

Olivia, age twenty-seven, is a very attractive woman. Even so, she rarely washes her hair and wears soiled clothes. Though she is a gifted painter, she never lets anyone see her work. When asked why, she says, "No one would believe that someone as ugly as I am could paint beautiful watercolors."

Sam is described by his teachers as "near perfect." But his divorced parents think otherwise. "He eats too much candy and is a sleepyhead," his mother says. "And sometimes he digs his little fingernails into the skin until he draws blood when he is hugging someone good-bye."

Are these classic examples of split personalities? Are Ben and young Sam displaying a Jekyll and Hyde syndrome? How can Olivia be so talented and so sick at the same time?

Ben, Olivia, and Sam are my clients. When we began working together, each was under the hypnotic spell of that part of them that has no conscience, disavows God, and creates pathological disorders in the lives of otherwise normal people. Each one manifested characteristics of ego manipulation and control. I'm happy to report that Ben and Olivia and Sam got better when they realized that their egos could, like an imp, cause trouble and even ruin their lives.

## What Is the Ego?

The ego is not an evil entity to be destroyed or avoided but a valuable aspect of us that needs to be reeducated. Unconscious and without boundaries, the ego is the part of us that mediates between the world and our natural human appetites for food, love, self-esteem, sexual gratification, intellectual stimulation, and companionship. Problems arise because the ego, while on a worthy mission, has no sense of proportion. It has a tendency to say things like, "You want a cookie? How about a whole box? Why stop at one glass of wine when you can drink every drop you can get your hands on?" Unleavened by our higher nature, ego lacks the moral and the spiritual forces that add balance and proportion to our lives. Ego on its own will not acknowledge itself as part of the larger whole, which demands fairness, sharing, balance, harmony, and community.

The idea that the ego is a sinister part of ourselves has been enhanced by many religions, which make self-annihilation the goal of spiritual growth and unfoldment. The path of self-annihilation may work for those who intend to live their lives sheltered from everyday realities, in the confines of ashrams or monasteries, but for the rest of us, nothing could be more impractical. We are trying to make our way in the material world and still be spiritual beings.

How can we accomplish this?

The answer is with an ego that stays in proportion to a healthy conscience. The first techniques I suggest to bring you into balance with your ego are visualization and dialogue. They help to reach a part of yourself that has been hidden from you for much of your life. While you have been out in the open and held accountable for your actions, your ego has been in hiding. Although your ego has been at the bottom of the things you've done, he has not been held accountable because to everyone but you he is silent and invisible.

I encourage clients to conceptualize the ego not only as shadow but also as a twin self. The thoughts and actions of both you and your ego create all of your negative and positive qualities.

## Visualization and Dialogue Exercise

First close your eyes. See yourself opening your arms as you would to greet a friend. Now embrace your ego, the mischief-maker who is stirring up all the trouble in your life. You may see your ego as all your defects and uncontrolled appetites rolled into one. After your embrace, step apart and ask ego to sit down. Just as if he were an actual person, talk with him. Let him know that you are not absolving yourself for your difficulties, and you need him to face your character defects with you.

The talk might go something like this:

You: "We're in a mess, you and I. What's going on?"

Ego: "I didn't get what I wanted. I wanted to do what I wanted to do when I wanted to do it. No controls. No limits. I encouraged you to eat and drink and buy what you wanted, go where you wanted, and not have to pay for a thing. I even showed you how to treat others so they would know who was boss. What's the problem?"

You: "The problem is obvious. Each person needs to live in balance and in sanity, so they can hear God's voice when He speaks. You're not mentioning how afraid I became because of you, not to mention the hundreds of shameful things we did together.

Moving in the middle of the night to avoid creditors or always having to make new friends because we drove the ones we had away."

Ego: "You weren't happy with the way things were, were you?"

You: "First, we are going to believe it's possible to change. No situation is hopeless unless we adopt a pessimistic outlook or decide to become a permanent victim. Second, God will help us if we ask Him to. The universe is good and He is our source. We've been hoodwinking ourselves all our lives and now it is time to take our spirit back."

Ego: "What if I don't like living the way you are suggesting?"

You: "God will refund your misery."

Ego: "Him? How do you know He will want me back?"

You: "Ego, if He's taken me, he'll take you."

Ego: "I'm afraid that just saying His name will kill me."

You: "I'll help you. Let's start by spelling it. Here we go together. . . ."

You and Ego: "G-O-D. God."

This dialogue bears the hallmarks of a healthy conversation with the ego. First, it's friendly. We don't get anywhere by beating ourselves up. The process of transformation begins with self-acceptance. Second, it's effective. Some people believe it takes forever to get back into God's graces. However, it is amazing how quickly things begin to turn around when you feel that your ego and you are aligned in purpose. My clients have testified to this fact. One client recently commented, "I never had a clue that somebody with my checkered past could feel so free once I stopped blaming my ego and cleaned up my act."

Finally, this sample dialogue between self and ego is transformative. Once there is a true coming to terms with the ego, many people experience a breakthrough. Coming to honest terms with self is the first step in the spiritual experience, just as the caterpillar must crawl into a cocoon before becoming a butterfly. When you confront your ego, you can have a happier, freer life.

## Ben, Olivia, and Sam

Fortunately Ben, Olivia, and Sam were able to break through the defense mechanisms of their egos. After two years of intense private therapy that included hypnosis regression—coming to terms with having been physically abused by his stepmother as a child—Ben eventually repaired his marriage with couples counseling. The piece of therapy that caused the biggest shift was when Ben realized that his stepmother had been abused herself and she did to him what had been done to her. Not only did he alter his thinking, but he also healed through identifying his character defect with hers. Ben learned how to communicate with his wife and children, and scheduled downtime for himself.

Olivia's self-esteem emerged through regular guided meditations centered on self-healing. She made a choice to accept her past and not let it paralyze her capacity to find happiness in her life. One day during her meditation, she remembered her mother shaming her with criticism, "You're wasting your time, missy. You'll never be a painter." Olivia found the courage to let her mother know that it was not okay for her to have treated Olivia as she did. Once Olivia discovered her worth, she paid attention to her appearance and also began to paint every day.

Sam needed a father substitute in order to learn to value himself. Without the guidance of a male role model, Sam was unable to feel good about himself or to get along with other children—he felt he was different and an outcast. After joining Big Brothers and being nurtured by a twenty-five-year-old man, he gradually developed the confidence to face what had caused his anger since infancy: His father had abandoned him and hence Sam felt that made him unworthy and less than his peers. He was able to express himself because there was a caring adult man to listen to him and offer suggestions on how to see himself as worthy of being loved.

Each of the three—Ben, Olivia, and Sam—had to confront the devil that chased him or her and turn ego into an angel who had come to help.

## Negative and Positive Qualities

Now that you are talking with your ego, reaching out to a part of yourself that has long been scolded or hidden, what are the negative qualities you are going to address? Remember, the process of confronting your ego involves brutal honesty. I invite you to compile a complete list of grievances from the wide range of compulsions and addictions listed below. Because I want you to have a balanced picture of yourself, be sure to compile a list of positive qualities, too, from the examples.

Take out a piece of paper and create a picture of who you are.

## Negative Qualities

| | | |
|---|---|---|
| Fearful | Alcoholic | Paranoid |
| Deceitful | Selfish | Self-centered |
| Overspending | Profligate | Wasteful |
| Sexually addicted | Manipulative | Gluttonous |
| Greedy | Jealous | Controlling |
| Impatient | Narcissistic | Envious |
| Gossipy | Passive-aggressive | Slothful |
| Distrustful | Angry | Vulgar |
| Physically abusive | Hateful | Stingy |

| Workaholic | Revengeful | Judgmental |
| Critical | Perfectionistic | Resentful |
| Vain | Arrogant | Dishonest |
| Cheater | Grandiose | Self-righteous |
| Pompous | Proud | Guilty |
| Self-loathing | Lustful | Two-faced |
| Covetous | Lazy | Self-seeking |
| Depressive | Possessive | Extravagant |

## Positive Qualities

| Faithful | Accepting | Conciliatory |
| Trustworthy | Loyal | Complimentary |
| Honest | Friendly | Positive |
| Frugal | Decent | Humble |
| Moderate | Industrious | Appeasing |
| Cooperative | Calm | Open |
| Generous | Loving | Giving |
| Flexible | Balanced | Gracious |
| Trusting | Generous | Joyful |
| Patient | Sharing | Comforting |
| Modest | Reliable | Responsible |
| Sensitive | Compassionate | Empathetic |

When you have created a portrait of yourself from the lists above, sit quietly for a few minutes. Next imagine all of your defects being released as pink balloons. In your mind's eye see the positive qualities as four-leaf clovers in a patch of grass and pick them one by one. Repeat this exercise once a week and over time you will see the positive results of your visualization. This technique is a form of subtle self-hypnosis or autosuggestion.

## Seek Out the Help You Need

In the process of unmasking and befriending your ego, seek help from a good friend or counselor if you don't want to go it on your own. And, of course, talk to people who know you and love you. You are not alone. The resources for dealing with whatever is keeping you from living the life God intended for you are without limits.

A dialogue with a friend might go something like this:

*You:* "I am too judgmental. What's wrong with me?"

*Friend:* "Nothing. Absolutely nothing. You expect too much of yourself."

*You:* "What do you mean?"

*Friend:* "High expectations cause all of us to act out with addictive behavior. Being harsh and critical is what your ego uses to keep you stirred up."

*You:* "What can I do to let go of this defect? It is driving me crazy."

*Friend:* "Do what I do. Keep a journal. Get it on paper and out of your head. Talk to your ego—the culprit. Reason with it. Treat him like a friend you've had a falling out with. Like you and I are having this conversation, let your ego know that you are doing the best you can with what you've got left, that you want to live and let live, and that you desire to accept yourself and others as doing the best you and they can do. And tell your ego a joke or two. All of us need to learn to laugh at ourselves."

When you talk with friends about your ego and your shortcomings, refer to ego as a close friend without whom your life would be incomplete. Two pilgrims—you and your ego—must walk hand-in-hand on God's path.

*Keep a Journal*

As you and your ego listen to what God has to say, you will live under a seal of cooperation. But what's next? How do you deal with life after you've made peace with your ego? How do we insure that we don't slip back into egocentric thinking?

The first thing that you might want to do is keep a journal. If you used one while learning how to meditate, continue to use it to monitor ego deflation. Writing your thoughts down gives you a new perspective on them, and you may be surprised at the insights you will gain from the simple exercise of journaling.

Here are some samples shared by my clients:

## April 16, 1993

I missed my meditation this morning and I paid for it with a very scattered day. No one seemed to want to give me what I thought I deserved—or maybe this "poor little ole me" attitude resurfaced. I will pray for God to help me achieve better discernment.

## July 4, 1993

I must remember that I cannot do a week's worth of work in a day. Staying at the office until ten o'clock at night is insanity. Tomorrow I am going to review my workload with my supervisor.

## November 23, 1993

I am going home for Thanksgiving, which means being around my sister, who always tries to goad me about still being single. She may try to talk about my weight problem being the reason that I am not married. To be able to remain still in my power I am going to talk to her before the family gathers to tell her how I feel about her criticism of me. She may say disparaging things to me anyway, but I will have spoken my truth. I meditated, wrote in my journal, and got to bed at a decent hour.

### Books

In addition to journaling, I recommend a lot of books to my clients. One of my favorites is *It's Not What You're Eating, It's What's Eating You* by Janet Greeson. Ms. Greeson is described as a diet guru, but her book is about more than food problems. It is also about changing the perception you have about yourself. She suggests that eating too little or too much is a problem. Her book guides you to find the source of your troubles so you can get in balance.

Another one of my favorites is M. Scott Peck's book *People of the Lie,* which offers insights into how to deal with lying, manipulation, narcissism, and the transference of defects from parents to their children.

### Prayer

Finally, the Serenity Prayer has helped millions of people hang on to hope until they were able to let God heal whatever afflicted them:

God, grant me the serenity to accept the things I cannot change, courage to change the things I can and wisdom to know the difference.

## Checklist for Deflating the Ego

1. Coax the ego with love and self-acceptance.

2. Talk with your ego through creative visualization.

3. Identify your negative and positive qualities.

4. Persist with autosuggestion until your ego cooperates.

5. Talk to trusted friends and seek professional help.

6. Keep a progress journal.

## Today and Every Day

Get up every day and greet your ego: "Friend, how do you feel? Do we need to resolve any unfinished business?"

Let him know how much you need his cooperation not only to make it through the day but also to be happy. You must live life together.

Follow the guidelines I have given you. The most important thing to remember, as the Hopi Indians suggest, is that "we die every night and are reborn every morning." The same is true for you and your shadow, your ego. You must reaffirm and reconnect every day for the rest of your life.

CHAPTER 21

# Your Family as Mirror

NO MATTER WHO WE ARE or what we do with our lives, nearly all our traits, good and bad, can be traced back to the family we grew up in. In essence, we become what we experience from the elders in our tribe.

Genetics certainly determine some of our traits, such as blue eyes, but so much of how we behave is the result of nurture, which combines everything we absorb from the people who raise us.

Now that we've integrated our ego, we need to take a look at the culture of our family. There is a premise often bantered about in psychology circles that if you want to know what's right or wrong with someone, get invited to dinner with their relatives. Both the good and bad traits will come toppling out of the proverbial family tree. Once we know what's in the tree, we can make changes in what we are growing and the fruit we pick.

Let's closely inspect your family tree. We have to start with an examination of where the good and bad seeds are planted. There is no better way to sort the rotten from the ripe in your family than to conduct an honest and fearless inventory. It's not just the bad stuff we're looking for here, we also need to know what's worth hanging on to in our family system.

## A Family Review

What was your family like? Were they secretive? Did your parents show favoritism? Was either of your parents narcissistic? Did you grow up feeling rejected or manipulated or abandoned? Or were your parents loving and nurturing? It is important to examine these attributes of family behavior to discover who you are—a well-balanced adult or a damaged soul. As you go through a review of the major family cultures listed below, take notes. For example, when you read about the secrecy-family culture, write about your own family secrets. If an unmarried aunt committed suicide after an abortion, don't relegate it to just another skeleton in the closet. Talk about it among family members and find out what emotion was at work—was the family guilty or ashamed? And why? In working with clients I find that those who write about everything without censorship get freer, faster.

### Negative Family Cultures

1. If your family was secretive . . .

Secrecy buries destructive patterns of distrust deep within the subconscious. Like a spider web, the nature of secrecy traps the ones keeping secrets so they can never be free of the implications of the covert information. For instance, if a father confides to his son that he has a mistress, the secret very often becomes the spawning ground for the son to be unfaithful to his wife when he marries. Go back and recall any family secrets that may be affecting your ability to be open and honest.

2. If your family showed favoritism . . .

Favoritism in the family circle devalues those who are not seen to be special, often producing a sense of inferiority. Favoritism often leads the neglected to seek approval from others as opposed to finding self-approval. And problems also occur in the favored ones. In *Silently Seduced: When Parents Make Their Children Partners: Understanding Covert Incest*, Dr. Kenneth M. Adams suggests that a daughter treated as daddy's little girl will be incapable of valuing her husband or developing a strong trusting bond with him. Adams views psychological, covert seduction of a girl by her father as the root cause of her inability to make a loving marriage with her husband. He writes, "I often advise such a daughter to divorce her father, not her husband."

Were you a favorite with a parent or was a brother or sister preferred? Get after the emotion before it robs you of any more joy.

3. If there was narcissism in your family . . .

Narcissism on the surface seems to be a character flaw of craving attention, but it more accurately describes a person who must live in a carefully constructed world that is a proxy for the person who needs to be examined and healed. For example, a narcissistic parent may encourage her children to look good on the outside but not foster positive traits on the inside. M. Scott Peck believes that narcissists are people constitutionally incapable of being honest with themselves or anyone else. They cannot accept blame of any kind and engage in constant scapegoating. Narcissistic people are self-absorbed, and often self-loathing. Do you identify with this trait? Was either of your parents afflicted with narcissism? Clear your feelings about how that trait made you feel.

4. If there was rejection in your family . . .

A rejected child has not been embraced with sufficient love and affection. Rejection affects a child's future as much as anything because he or she feels unworthy of love or success. The primary damage seems to be one's inability to succeed in a relationship or career, though rejection can also penetrate to the core of an individual's self-worth with devastating results. Parents or other supervising adults who live in a materialistic world tend to reject children based upon their intelligence, popularity, looks, and social skills, and lack thereof. If you felt rejected as a child, get in touch with those feelings. You can always talk about these feelings with a counselor or trusted friend or minister.

## Barry's Story

Barry came from a family where everyone talked at once. His mother was always trying to be a referee rather than a mother: "Sarah, come back here and finish your breakfast. Sam, stop picking on your sister. And don't forget you have a dentist appointment at four o'clock. Barry, be home right after school. I need you to cut the grass."

Barry's father would come home at night extremely tired with very little to say except to make demands. "I don't want to hear about anything from any of you. I've had a hard day. Just shut up and leave me alone. I already give you everything under the sun."

"Father definitely did not 'know best' at my house," Barry said. "It was his way or the highway. It was so bad that I thought about walking out and never coming back."

The solution for Barry's parents was to give their children everything money could buy—but not discipline, nurturing, and the time to communicate. Barry was not sure whether he was living in Grand Central Station or in his house—there was always so much racket he couldn't hear himself think. The one thing that was obvious to him was that his boisterous family members were each going in a different direction.

One day Barry, age seventeen, had a bright idea. If no one could hear anybody else speak because they were too busy talking, he'd write each member of the family a letter. Here's a sample of what he wrote:

Dear Dad:

I know your job is rough and you are tired when you get home. However, all of us are busy and have no time for anyone else, but we are making it worse by not communicating with one another. I am trying to graduate from high school with grades good enough to get into a good school on full scholarship. I think I'm smart enough, but what I need is a dad to talk to about what's going on with me. I'd like some help with where to apply to school, what to major in, how to handle girls, *when* to open my own checking account, and a lot of other things which you know better than I. Also, I get the idea all the time that you and Mother don't care about your kids. There are no rules; we don't have curfews and it seems like you expect teachers and Sunday School teachers and the preacher to be our conscience.

So here's what I propose: Every Saturday morning at ten o'clock we sit down together as a family and go over what's going on in our lives. The only rule is that one person speaks at a time. Not only do we talk about what's going on, but how we feel about any and everything inside the family. I hope that you and Mother will be open to changing your minds about being more like real parents to us.

Love,
Barry

It didn't happen overnight, but Barry got a powwow going and the family began learning how to hear and to listen to one another. Not only did Barry's family learn to share their true feelings, but also his parents reexamined what they needed to change to become better parents.

5. If there was manipulation in your family . . .

If a parent tries to force his will onto a child with little or no regard for the child's wishes, the child's repressed rage can cause problems later. Manipulation can also cause irreparable damage that results in a child growing up incapable of making decisions. Many clients tell me how they have a hard time making up their mind about the most inconsequential matters because of a manipulative mother or father. Manipulation often causes emotional paralysis. Were you manipulated as a child? How are you dealing with it now?

6. If there was sexual abuse in your family . . .

Sexual abuse is one of the most damaging of all family patterns. A child needs love and a safe environment to learn how to have sound relationships of a platonic and a romantic nature. Sexual abuse starts a pathological cycle for the child in which he may eventually become a perpetrator. It also robs the child of trust in dealing with others and plants seeds of self-loathing and difficulty in bonding. Were you sexually abused as a child? Who was the perpetrator? Have you ever discussed this with anyone? Buried anger can lead to depression. There are many qualified counselors to help you work through these feelings.

7. If there was abandonment in your family . . .

Abandonment triggers a sense of fear and loathing of the outside world. A child subjected to an environment in which he feels no one is there to love, guide, and teach him about life will create his own isolated world. Abandonment creates the orphan mentality. Did you feel abandoned as a child? How have you compensated? Do you know now that you are not alone?

### Positive Family Cultures

Looking at the destructive aspects of the family system is only one half of the equation. It's also important to look at the positive patterns and traits. They are your family's most precious heirlooms.

1. If your family was nurturing . . .

If your parents loved and supported you emotionally, your life as an adult rests on a firm foundation. Nurturance is one of the most important qualities to be found in the home environment. Were you nurtured as a child? Did your parents show love and affection to you and your siblings?

2. If your family used reasonable discipline . . .

Children who are given reasonable rules and regulations are more likely to grow up to be better adjusted and loving. Being raised without boundaries creates chaos in a child's life. Families with absentee parents foster greater risks of alcohol and drug abuse among children. Dedicated and hands-on parenting does not involve physical abuse but rather sensible rules. Did your family have house rules and benchmarks for you to try to reach? How did you react to discipline?

3. If your family was rich in parental involvement . . .

If parents are part of a child's life, it makes him feel they care. If a parent's work schedule precludes his being involved in activities of importance to the child, the child must be made to understand why the parent was not there and, perhaps, a surrogate can stand in whenever possible. Dr. Frank S. Pittman's book *Man Enough: Fathers, Sons and the Search for Masculinity,* discusses the importance of a father's participation in his son's life, especially when the boy reaches puberty and adolescence. It is a book that can aid the reader in rethinking what masculinity means to him. Were your parents actively involved in your life? Did you sense that they were doing all they could to support you and your activities?

4. If your family were good communicators . . .

The lack of understanding between parents and their children often occurs because the family does not sit down to discuss problems. A set time for family meetings improves the chances that misunderstandings find peaceful solutions. If a father speaks directly to his son or daughter in a family meeting, discussion flows unfiltered. Clearing the air at least once a week keeps the family on the same frequency. Did your family discuss things openly? Did you feel that you were listened to and heard?

5. If your family had a spiritual core . . .

In my experience, families that have a spiritual philosophy seem to have fewer incurable problems. Adopting an open-door policy allows the children to choose their own spiritual or religious path as they get older and builds acceptance and trust between parents and child. Did you have an active religious or spiritual life when you were growing up? Did you feel that you were free to follow your heart in this area after you were an adult?

6. If your family was open and honest . . .

When a child grows up feeling that there are no family secrets to undermine his sense of trust, he is able to meet the world with openness and integrity. Full disclosure in all matters ensures calmer waters and stronger character as the child matures. Has honesty been a problem in your family? Did you trust your parents? Were you trustworthy?

## Acknowledging Your Role in the Family

Once you have an understanding of the qualities that describe your family system, you can claim your part in what went wrong and what went right. Begin by making a list of all family members, starting with yourself.

1. You
2. Mother
3. Father
4. Siblings
5. Grandparents
6. Other significant family members (aunts, uncles)

Now for the difficult part. Will you take responsibility for harming anyone in your family? The harm can be mental, emotional, or financial. It can be about character assassination (gossip), dishonesty in relationships (extramarital affairs or unfaithful to a lover), or being unloving with deeds and words with our parents, siblings, spouses, and children. This exercise reveals a lot about what triggers you emotionally and psychologically.

Do you see yourself in any of the following examples?

1. My father favored my sister, so I always tried to undermine her.

2. My father made me eat foods I didn't like, so I channeled my anger at his manipulation into my relationship with my younger brother.

3. My mother kept secrets, so I learned to hide the whole truth from my husband.

4. Nobody in my family ever listened to one another, so I find my wife and kids and I talk all at once.

5. I was a latchkey kid, so I find it hard to make friends for fear they will leave me.

6. My daughter has a tendency to procrastinate in all areas of her life—just like I do—so I catch myself being unduly hard.

Once you have identified your harmful actions, you can pray for the people you have harmed. And don't forget to pray for the strength and wisdom to be gentle with yourself during this fearless inventory.

I'd like to give the last word in this chapter to medical intuitive Caroline Myss, whose book *Why People Don't Heal and How They Can*, discusses the language of "woundology," a term she coined to describe people whose entire life is stuck in what happened to them in childhood. Myss tells a story about a woman who talks endlessly about having been an incest victim when someone asks her a simple question. When the therapist to whom she was speaking asked how long ago, the woman answered, "Thirty years. I remember it as if it were yesterday."

Myss says that if you don't heal the past, you will never live in the present.

Remember, if you spend your entire life licking wounds, that's victimhood. You must do the best you can to make your life better, accept the things you cannot change, and move on. Life should not be an endless dig for skeletons of the past but an expression of the joy of living.

# CHAPTER 22

# Remembering Who You Really Are

*"To thine own self be true, and then it must follow
as the day the night, thou canst not then be false to
any man."*
—Shakespeare

It seems that since the day we were born, someone has been telling
us who we are, what to do, and what is expected of us. Many parents
start picking out their kid's college the minute he or she is born.
From the cradle to college and beyond, our life is very often not our
own.

Many fathers expect their sons to follow their career path, and if
the father establishes control and dominance early enough, the son
won't stand a chance to break out of dad's clutches.

Mothers can be even more dominating with daughters. "Dear,
you must pledge my sorority." "You're dating whom? Is he one of *the*
Wilsons from Montecito?" "Nice girls don't do that, so you can forget about going." In the South, we call proper young ladies magnolia
blossoms, because they look so sweet and pretty. Whispered rumor
has it that Magnolia can be quite deadly if she successfully learns all
of Momma's tricks.

## Jarrod's Story

Jarrod was a very successful surgeon practicing in Palm Beach, Florida. He had gone to all the right schools, joined the right clubs, and had married his beautiful childhood sweetheart. Jarrod had two sons whom he doted on and was living in a mansion on the ocean. Living the life of Riley? Yes. Was he happy? Absolutely not.

In going over his discontent with a counselor he discovered that he had done everything his father expected of him: He went to the schools his father picked, joined his father's clubs, and married a girl his father liked. And his father, also a surgeon, had badgered Jarrod from childhood to go to medical school.

"What did *you* want to do with your life?" the counselor asked Jarrod.

"I always wanted to live in the hills of Virginia, not on the beach in Florida. I want to raise horses as well as own and operate a bed-and-breakfast. Surgery is not where my passion is. I might like to teach at a small private school. These are the things I have wanted to do my whole life."

Not only was Jarrod not living his passion, he was living his father's idea of what his life should be. It took him three years, but Jarrod finally moved to Virginia after his father died unexpectedly. But why should he have had to wait for his father's death to be able to do and be who and what he wanted?

## Identifying Controlling Forces

Being ourselves—instead of fulfilling the hopes, wishes, and dreams of our parents, teachers, preachers, and friends—starts by identifying where the control over us began. Examine the following list to see if you can identify with some of the examples of manipulation and domination by parents, authority figures, and friends.

1. My parents never asked me where I wanted to go to school.

2. My father made me play soccer and football because he liked the sports.

3. My teacher told me I should teach, like her.

4. My friends told me who was "in" or "out" at school.

5. My preacher said I should marry someone of my own faith.

6. My father wouldn't let me take dance lessons; he said it was for sissies.

7. My parents sent me to the same summer camp they went to.

8. Mother said that I should wear certain clothes because they were preppy.

9. Dad told me I should go to law school.

10. My parents made me go to church every Sunday.

11. My father discouraged me from going to the opera. "It's not manly," he would say.

12. My parents told me, "This family votes only Republican!"

If these examples have made you realize that those dearest to you are your biggest deterrent to self-realization, don't despair. It is never too late to correct a mistake. For instance, if your mother talked you into taking a job that doesn't suit you, consider making a change. Change doesn't need to be abrupt or dramatic. You can proceed slowly if you wish. Go back to school. Get retrained. Or be a self-starter. Have a great idea for a business? Become an entrepreneur. Whatever you do, don't blame your mother for the choice you made. Take responsibility to change the things you can.

Go back to that place in life where you took a turn left and you would rather have gone right. Was it when you didn't take a course of study you really wanted? Did you marry before you had a chance to live your dream of becoming. . . . You fill in the blank. It's never too late to become whomever and whatever you were going to be and do when you grew up. It only takes sacrifice and risk.

Did you know that sacrifice and risk put together is a sacred dare? That's right. If you decide that you can live your dream by waking up from your nightmare, you will be taking a divine chance to become who you really are.

## Culture as a Controlling Force

Parents, other family, and friends are not the only culprits we've allowed to control our lives, although as our role models they are accountable for the pressure cookers they put us in. Let's take a look now at how our pervasive popular culture has asserted its power over our life choices.

Driven by advertisers who influence what we wear, what and where we eat, how we spend our dollars and on what, our personal choices are lost in a mudslide of hidden and overt persuaders. There is a popular sociology that speaks of the herd mentality. We may recognize the herd mentality as "keeping up with the Joneses." And in this herd thinking, there is very little room for personal choice.

All the advertising hype makes it more difficult to steer clear of a stampede of peer pressure and do what feels right for you. For instance, an actor plays a character in a film that is advertised and marketed incessantly. You respond to the hype and go see the film, where you fall in love with the character's perfect life. You want to be the character for whom everything works out. And the spin-off products of the film—designer jeans and sunglasses—are telling you that you can be, with this purchase. No wonder you can't leave the character in the theatre after the show! When you begin to look like, dress like, and act like a movie actor, you need to take a good look at your values.

To get to the heart and soul of who you are, you need to pull out of the foray of media madness and pop culture. If you are ever going to be happy, a housecleaning to decide what you can throw out of your life is necessary. I ask my clients to tell me in one sentence what they want. Here are some of the answers.

1. I want to turn my life over to God.
2. I want to eat healthier and get plenty of rest.
3. I want happiness that isn't based on money.
4. I want to travel, not save a fortune.
5. I want to prioritize learning and discovering.
6. I want to live without concern for wardrobe and fancy cars.
7. I want to write and paint.
8. I want to visit a new country every year.
9. I want to do something to help others.
10. I want to laugh more and worry less.

So many people tell me that they thought that a new car, a new house, stylish clothes, or an exotic vacation would satisfy them. A few weeks after getting all of these things, they felt empty again. Self-satisfaction is an inside job. You can enjoy life, but the peace that you seek is to be found in our inner world—rarely outside yourself.

### Controlling Forces of Church and State

We have all given an inordinate amount of our power away to church and state in our culture. I say it's time to keep your faith and vote your conscience; live your truth. Too much of what we think and how we act is based on who is the biggest bully or can shout the loudest or evoke the most guilt or attempt to speak for God. Steer clear of any platform that tries to cast your vote for you or an agenda that interprets what God would have you do. These choices are your own. Make them.

## How to Gain Self-Perspective Among All the Noise

A clean break from the influences of family, friends, culture, church, and state can be aided and abetted by a silent weekend. You don't need to go to a monastery or retreat center, although they can enhance the process. Simply be alone and be quiet. Next write a wish list for how you would like to see your life from now on.

On a sheet of paper, build two columns. Label column one, What I Was Told to Do, and column two, What I Told Myself to Do. This is a good assessment of whose life are you living: your own or your parents', authority figures', a spouses', or a friend's? For example:

| I Was Told . . . | I Told Myself . . . |
|---|---|
| Where to go to school | Who I should marry |
| What to major in | When to start a family |
| What job to take | What faith I would follow |
| What city was best | Who I would vote for |
| What insurance to buy | What I valued in a friend |

This exercise will also help you to uncover what you stand for and what counts the most with you. To reinforce what you stand for and begin to lead a transformed life, I suggest following these tenets:

1. I am willing to sacrifice luxuries to be able to live my passion rather than to work at something I don't enjoy.

2. I am willing to live and let live regarding other people's religious beliefs, but I do not want anyone telling me what and how to believe.

3. I am willing to take an annual housecleaning of what I want for my life as opposed to what I am settling for, and to take the steps necessary to make positive changes.

4. I am willing to see what I can do for others rather than to live selfishly.

5. I am willing to work on my character to make sure that I am considered trustworthy, ethical, and tolerant rather than a self-centered materialist.

6. I am willing to turn my will and my life over to God every day.

When you make new game rules and play by them, you uncover your authentic self and live a life that you have worked diligently to create. Letting go of the defended self—which by definition is not the real you but a creation of someone else—permits you to live life with unlimited joy and peace of mind. You can have this richer life if you will live by your own rules.

Starting over can be risky and can be a divine dare. Dare to live with authenticity and clarity about who you are and what you want to create in your life. Read and discover worlds that were once only in encyclopedias or required reading. Go on vacations that make your world larger. Value that which is worthless to so many people in the world but priceless to you.

## Dorothy's Story

The one thing Dorothy determined to do when she finished college was travel and see places she had only read about. With a hefty inheritance from her grandparents, she set out for the Greek Islands on the first leg of an around-the-world tour.

In Greece, she fell in love with a native named Nicholas and quickly married him. Nick wanted to move to the United States, so Dorothy gave up her dream to roam. She settled down and started a family.

When the last of her three children left for college, Dorothy had just turned forty-five. Her investments had paid off handsomely, and she decided that she wanted to take that long-delayed trip around the world. There was one thing stopping her. Nicholas had a business to run and couldn't join Dorothy for a yearlong vacation. What was she to do? Give up her trip because her husband couldn't go? In a quiet moment she was inspired with a solution.

"Nicholas, you still own some property on Santorini. How would you like to build a house there and live here in the United States for six months and there, six months each year?"

"But, Dorothy, I have a business to run."

"Sell it."

"Sell it? Who would want to buy it? What if I don't get what it's worth?

"Who cares? We have more than enough money to last us a lifetime—even if we both live to be 100. Let's do it."

After a series of discussions, to Dorothy's surprise, Nicholas agreed.

And so they built a house in Greece and lived six months there and six months in the United States each year. Nicholas opened an import-export business and Dorothy became a boutique travel guide for destinations all over the world.

"We won't have a closely knit group of friends and the kids will have to come a long way for us to baby-sit, but I am living the life I always wanted to live," Dorothy told one of her travelers.

Was Dorothy being selfish? Nicholas, in the end, didn't think so. Life involves compromise. For many years, she had lived her husband's life. And, for the price of asking—for daring to ask—she finally got to live the life she desired with her husband's blessings.

# CHAPTER 23

# Practicing Forgiveness

ANDY GREW UP IN A TYPICAL middle-class family. He was quiet and studious and pleasant to be around. He made good grades, was active in student government, and acted in school plays. When someone got angry with Andy, he would skulk away. When a teacher falsely accused him of cheating, he nodded a half-hearted denial and took a walk. And when his father showed favoritism to his younger brother, Andy didn't seem to mind.

When he graduated from college, Andy got a coveted professional position in medical research in Boston. Everything was going smoothly for Andy until a colleague was promoted into a job Andy wanted. Although he said nothing, he began to call in sick. Coworkers noticed he was gaining a considerable amount of weight. After being warned repeatedly about absenteeism, Andy was fired.

Andy was fired from five more jobs in less than ten years. He was never able to stay in a relationship because he would throw violent tantrums and sob uncontrollably when things didn't go his way. His weight continued to balloon and he started drinking and smoking.

A therapist worked with Andy for months before any explanation came out of him. Andy started talking about the upsets he had been holding inside of him, which went back to his childhood.

"Kids at school made fun of me because I always struck out in ball games; Miss Sidelman, my tenth-grade algebra teacher, falsely accused me of cheating on an examination; I believed that my father loved my brother, Eric, much more than he did me. How would that make you feel? I never felt that anybody cared if I lived or died."

Andy kept working with his counselor until he dug up all the buried bones of his youth. He healed because he was not only able to get in touch with his hidden anger, but he also dismantled his resentments. The word *resent* literally means to feel something over and over again. Andy was locked in his inner world, silently railing at his tormentors, one of whom was his father.

At the center of Andy's maelstrom was a fear so paralyzing that it actually kept him in bed—fear was the source of his being fired for not showing up at work. The reason he was unable to diffuse the fear was because he had been ridiculed so much in his life that he did not want to admit that he was afraid. His counselor determined that Andy had panic attacks brought on by concealing his feelings under a pile of fear.

There is a relationship that can alter hurt feelings and give you the courage to take the steps to clean up what caused your anger and resentments: The relationship is with God. Anger and resentment keep most of us in a murky cloud that blocks God's voice. We cannot hear Him because we are holding on to something somebody said or something they did. That something can be only a slight, but it can seem huge in our minds. Anger builds. Resentments fester. We cannot let go of the harm we feel someone has done to us. The underbelly of anger is a fear of what might happen if we confront whomever we believe has done us wrong. Fear causes us to come out swinging in our heads, hearts, and minds, even when we don't address the problem in real life.

When we become aware of how angry we are with someone and

how we resent that person, we need to find a way to release the built-up pressure or we run the risk of blowing up.

## Writing Rage Letters

In Chapter 21 we made a list of those persons whom we had harmed and discussed who had harmed us. In order to purge your feelings, I want you to write letters of anger and rage to those persons who have harmed you. It is vital to empty out all of the pent-up feelings you have toward these persons. Even if something happened yesterday, use this method. You will not be sending these letters, so there is no need to censor yourself. Anger and rage letters are not meant to be sent; they are only an exercise to release stored anger.

Here's the one Andy wrote to his teacher:

Dear Miss Sidelman:

Although I have been out of your class for twenty years, I am still trapped in a prison of repressed rage at you because you falsely accused me of cheating. What did that incident do to my self-esteem? How did it affect my life? You'd have to read my résumé and talk to my therapist to know just how bad life has been for me.

I have hated you so much that I've wanted many times to come into your classroom and hit you. Do you know how hurtful it is to a sixteen-year-old to have his teacher shame him? I was not guilty. You said I looked guilty. Well, Miss Sidelman, I was born looking guilty but I was not and am not!

You may not change one bit from this letter, but I assure you that I will feel tons better for expressing how I really felt about what you did to me.

Sincerely,
Andy Sikes

## Writing Letters of Forgiveness to Others

After completing your anger and rage letters, it's time to write letters of forgiveness to the people who have harmed you. Through forgiveness, your hurt and anger will resolve itself. All of my clients agree that forgiveness is the way to clear up hurt feelings and to repair relationships.

Dear Miss Sidelman:

I was in your math class in 1967, and I wanted to write you a letter to make amends for my behavior. Although I like to think that I was a perfect kid in your class, I know if I am honest with myself, I was not.

I am going through a period of introspection and because of certain things that have come up in this process, I needed to write you this letter.

Miss Sidelman, if I did anything to make your role as a teacher more difficult, I wish to make amends to you. I cannot change what I may have done, but I can humble myself to ask for your forgiveness. Also, as an opportunity to make things better with you, I signed up to work with a young man in the Big Brother program. Perhaps I can make a difference with a teenager who is struggling like I did.

Sincerely,
Andy Sikes

## Seeking Forgiveness for Yourself

After you empty your soul of lingering resentments against those who have caused you injury and have written letters forgiving them, the next step is to seek forgiveness from those you have harmed.

We ought not to send letters initially to those we have victimized. They are exercises in finding closure for bad relationships that keep us from moving forward in our lives. Perhaps at a later date, when the effect of a letter has transformed its author, he or she may decide to make amends in person, or send a revised letter.

I always counsel letter writers to get quiet before starting the process of forgiveness. Meditate. Listen for that still, small voice to guide you from attachment to negative emotions to freedom from the bondage of self and others. Claiming your part in broken relationships or bad behavior will reconnect you to God more than any other action you take.

The repentant is strongly urged not to write, "I'm sorry," or "I apologize," for we have all been saying those empty and meaningless words all of our lives. Making amends means changing one's heart in order to make things better between two or more people.

Here is a forgiveness letter from a man named Adam. Adam's life took the same detours as those of his father: He is a twice-divorced alcoholic. This letter seeking forgiveness was his ticket to emotional and spiritual freedom:

Dear Dad:

I am in Sedona, Arizona, going through a powerful program of healing. After a week of facing years of resentments, anger, and rage, I was asked to write a letter of forgiveness to anyone I had harmed in my life. You were the first person I thought of. I needed to write you this letter.

The hook to a letter of forgiveness is that I must ask for your forgiveness rather than to expect you to seek my forgiveness. This was real hard at first, until I began to understand what forgiveness is: forgiving the part of myself that is you—that you represent.

When you and Mom divorced around my ninth birthday, I thought I had done something wrong. When money ran low and she had to work two jobs to support us kids, I thought it was my fault. When we heard you lost your job of over twenty-five years, I wondered what I could have done to prevent it. Why would I assume responsibility for all of these things when obviously none of it was my fault? I discovered through an honest inventory that I am selfish and self-centered. My taking responsibility for this stuff had a lot to do with thinking I should be able to make things better, when in essence it was God's business and none of mine.

We have to write about our family, which includes background information on you and Mom. As I started to reconstruct your childhood, I found out by talking to Grandmother that you had some difficult situations to work through. She said that you were born during the Depression and had to drop out of college in order to help the family financially. Grandmother said that there were no student loans and that Granddaddy retired early at half pension. Money was tight and it took you seven years to get your degree. You were an honor student and a top-flight debater. And you worked sixty hours a week for more than four years. I never knew any of this. Knowing you better helps me accept you as I had condemned you before.

You probably know that I have been married and divorced twice and have a daughter from one marriage and a son from the other. I swore I would never get divorced and yet I did—twice! Like father, like son?

Dad, I would probably never nominate you for father of the year and I have had a lot of years to regret your absence from my life, but this letter is about my amends to you. I never tried to find out how you were doing and I never sent a Father's Day card, called you on your birthday, or tried to see you at Christmas or any other holiday. I have never walked in your shoes and don't have a clue what kind of marriage you and Mom had. But I do know that I am choosing to make peace and start to have a relationship with you by asking for your forgiveness.

If I have ever said or done or failed to say or do anything that kept you from God's love and light, I ask you to forgive me. To make amends I am going to ask God to bless your life, to give you everything that I would ask for myself. And from this day forth until I die, I will always love and support you, and will speak of you only in loving terms. I am going to encourage my children to get to know you. Brother Bill and I want to ask you to go fishing in Minnesota this summer. Yes, Dad, we do remember the way it was before you and Mom split; just us three trying to land a ten pound bass or telling the biggest whopper about the one that got away.

You are my dad and I will always love you. Please forgive me.

Love,
Adam

Some letters are harder to write because of the nature of what happened between two people. But forgiveness is the only way I've found to get rid of the destructive, negative tie that binds one person to another. Forgiveness is not about endorsing someone's behavior or attempting to become more intimate with the perceived perpetrator. It is about getting out of the victim role and taking back our power. It's about releasing ourselves from the past so that we can truly thrive in the present.

Laura had been kidnapped, raped, and robbed while hiking through the jungles of Central America with her boyfriend, Jackson, who was also beaten and sexually assaulted. Left for dead, Laura and Jackson wandered aimlessly for three days before being found. When they returned home, Jackson swore Laura to secrecy about the sexual violations because he was so ashamed by what had happened.

Laura had an amends letter to write to Jackson. Remember that she had already unloaded all her pent-up rage against him with our therapists prior to writing this letter.

Dear Jackson:

Although fifteen years have passed since the kidnapping and assault, what happened to us all those years ago still festered inside me. At a healing retreat I have been facing buried shame and this incident needed to be uncovered and healed.

I have already raged at you. Your attitude toward what happened to us was reprehensible; some would even say unforgivable. But if I don't see my part in this I will be sixty years old someday, still emotionally paralyzed by the rape and brutality and your shoddy attitude about it.

Jackson, your family saw you as the fair-haired only son who was destined for great things. In your twenty-two-year-old mind, telling your mother and father and sisters about what happened would have branded you somehow less of a man. Our culture is so polarized and defensive about sexuality that perhaps there would have been a stigma. I never saw all of this as something that you couldn't do because of what others might think. I wanted to shout from the rooftop that I had been raped and left for dead. You wanted us to take a bath and forget it. And that's what we did.

I now see that you did the best you could under the circumstances and for those times. You were devastated and damaged as much as I was. For more than fifteen years I have been licking my wounds as if you had punished me for having been raped. I am the only one who can harm me by continuing to wage the war against you.

I am seeing what happened to us differently. In some

strange but unexplainable way, I know that you and I created this fiasco and we're the only ones who can heal it. I
have walked through the door of willingness to seek forgiveness and to stop letting the rape keep me stuck in the out-
back bleeding and dying and raging against you and those
teenage boys.

Please forgive me for trying to get you to see us as
poor, defenseless victims. I have come to see that drinking
all night in a bar wasn't the smartest thing we could have
done. Whatever you did, you did. We had three good
years as friends and lovers and I am going to let those
memories be lasting ones. You were powerless to lift the
lid on my grave of grief and heal it. Only I can do that and
I am.

Thank you for having been in my life and thank you for
my opportunity to look inside of me, where God and true
forgiveness live.

Sincerely,
Laura

## Practicing Forgiveness

When we look at how Laura could resolve the pain of Jackson's
abandonment and devaluation of her, we noticed that she kept saying how haunted she was by the rape and that she couldn't let go of
hurt feelings of shame. The forgiveness letter was but a first step in
clearing away the resentment she felt toward Jackson because he
had convinced her to deny that she had been raped. There was a
missing piece of the process of forgiveness.

Laura kept saying, "Something's stuck in my craw."

The dark cloud lifted when she went through transformational breath work with a licensed therapist here in Sedona.
Transformational breath work is the technique that allowed

Laura to release stored emotional trauma in her body and cellular memory through repetitive deep breathing, bringing fresh breath into areas that were holding trauma. Laura's body—as do all of ours—operates much like her subconscious, in that she had been unconsciously holding stress and trauma since the horrific rape.

When Laura's boyfriend silenced her, she stored the feelings and pain of what had happened, and without treatment these stored toxic feelings negatively affected her relationships with her husband, her children, her friends, and others with whom she dealt on a daily basis. Once she was able to resolve these destructive stored emotions, she was able to find peace and start to feel forgiveness of herself and Jackson.

In a transformational breath session, the patient lays down fully clothed on a table while music plays softly in the background. The practitioner intuits where the breathing is restricted. She gently guides the patient to open her breath in order to release the stagnant stored emotions. During the process, the practitioner asks the patient questions to access these stored traumatic memories.

"Did you have a traumatic episode with a family male figure when you were five?"

"Have you any memory of having been unduly upset with your brother or sister when you were a teenager?"

"Can you picture in your mind how you felt on that day in Central America when you were raped?"

The answers to these questions are revealed through a dramatic change in the rhythm of the breath, as well as crying, sobbing, and cries of rage. But it is in this emotional outpouring that the trauma is released.

Transformational breath work is available throughout the country.

*Keeping the Breath Clear and Living in Forgiveness*

Here are several suggested techniques for remaining clear of trauma and stored negative emotions in order to live in forgiveness:

1. Use breathing as a form of meditation. Monitor your breath. Follow this exercise for at least twenty minutes three times a week for a month.
2. Listen to soft music.
3. Get frequent massages.
4. Go to stretch classes, receive reflexology treatments, and work with a cranial sacral technician.
5. Practice yoga.
6. Develop a strong mind-body balance.
7. Journal your thoughts.
8. Go into grief counseling, if necessary.
9. Release resentments toward those who have harmed you.
10. Seek forgiveness from those who you have harmed.
11. Take a daily inventory, and when you are wrong, seek immediate forgiveness.

*A Happy Ending*

The forgiveness letter to Jackson started the healing process for Laura. The transformational breath work cleared up stored emotions and trauma associated with the rape. She continued suggested aftercare therapies to remain stress-free, which helped her to live in an attitude of forgiveness of herself and others.

Within six months, she enrolled in college at the age of forty-six to get the last ten hours of course work she needed to graduate. The communication with her family and friends became more direct but loving. She plans to open a retreat center for spiritual development for families on her 2,000-acre desert prairie. Laura now knows that healing happens when you learn to forgive and be forgiven.

PART IV

# The Power and Promise
# of the New Language

CHAPTER 24

# You, the Tuning Fork

I HAVE A CONFESSION TO MAKE. I was never a very good science student. Miss Walker taught me in tenth grade why a magnet draws metal to itself and how electricity travels from one lightning rod to another, but I only made a B— in her class. I didn't perform well in chemistry class in college either, but it was during that time that I came to understand that you can believe something without knowing exactly how it works. Instead of learning the intricacies of chemistry, I learned to become a person of strong faith.

Many of life's truths must be taken on faith. That's just the nature of human experience. When the authors of the Declaration of Independence wrote, "We hold these truths to be self-evident," they were acknowledging what they knew life should be about: liberty and the pursuit of happiness. Evidence doesn't give substance to truth. Truth has an absolute value that does not depend on standards of verification.

## The Nature of Thought

Thought is the most critical component of the new language. When we are quiet and still, God places His thought forms, or thought impressions, in our minds as a source of inspiration or instruction. These are the thoughts in our head that startle us. We say, "Where did that idea come from?" They are the thoughts that are distinctly not our own. When I was sitting in the back of a police car years ago, having been arrested for drinking and driving, the voice in my head that said, "It's over," was a thought impression from God.

Besides divine thought forms, our human minds, of course, also generate thought. Emanating from each one of us like vibrations from a tuning fork, thoughts are impulses of energy that send our joy and fear, judgments and criticisms, encouragement and dismay, anger, doubt, love, belief, and condemnation out into the universe. These emotional thoughts are powerful forces that can shape events and outcomes as a high-pitched voice can shatter glass. These thoughts are dynamic and influential—they affect the entire world. Although individual thought may not have a determining effect, it can serve as a strong contributing factor. If we have destructive thoughts, we are apt to create chaos. If we send out positive thoughts of peace, that possibility is manifested as well.

The creative nature of thought poses a choice. Will our thoughts be powerfully positive or destructively negative? Controlling our frame of mind is the issue. We can scrub our thoughts and alter what we are sending out to the universe, which I like to think of as recalibrating our human tuning fork. Or we can dump our hostility out into the world and potentially wreak havoc.

Emmet Fox was a strong advocate of constructive thinking. He gave his views about the vibrational universe we live in in his book *Make Your Life Worthwhile*. "You have doubtless seen and heard a tuning fork vibrating, thereby producing a certain note," Fox wrote. "Stop the vibration with your finger and the note ceases." What Fox seems to be suggesting is that we are able to stop negative thinking and alter the messages we are sending out before they contaminate. The shrill sound of the high-pitched tone need not reach the glass it has the power to shatter.

It makes sense to try to raise the positive vibration of our thoughts, but it is easier to say than to do. Having followed the same mental habits and mental diet for a lifetime, many of us are predisposed to a thinking style that may be the reflexive result of the environment in which we grew up. Some of us are pessimistic by upbringing; we are given to dark, ominous thoughts. Others are optimistic; we expect the best and look on the bright side, instinctively finding the positive in any given situation and dealing with problems constructively.

One useful exercise to find out how you think is to eavesdrop on yourself. Listening in on your internal conversations reveals a lot about who you are. You may discover that worry, dread, fear, jealousy, backbiting, and pessimism generally color most of your thoughts. Interestingly, a lot of these emotions are tied to dwelling in the past or in the future. On the other hand, you might find that you are generally happy, joyful, hopeful, accepting, loving, compassionate, and kind.

In addition to observing your thinking style, you gain self-knowledge by watching what might be called the time zone of thinking to see if you have a tendency to exist in the past, present, or future. Set aside a period of time in which you make it a priority to watch yourself thinking. Monitor your thoughts during this period and note where your attention is placed. Are you remembering and reliving something that happened in the past? Are you anticipating something coming up? Or are you paying attention to what is happening in the here and now?

In his book *The Power of Now*, Eckhart Tolle suggests that most people who try this exercise will be surprised at how much of their "mind-time" is in the future or past. Tolle believes that "the time-bound mode of our consciousness is deeply embedded in the human psyche" and that a period of great transformation will be ushered in when the mass consciousness begins to focus on the here and now. He further suggests that mental suffering and anxiety are largely a function of living in the past and in the future. Tolle advocates breaking the "mind patterns that have dominated human life for eons" by working to keep our minds oriented in the present, where we make it our goal to be constructive.

For most people this is a very difficult task. Most of us have been raised to treat thinking as a casual and control-free activity, not a conscious one. Except in meditation, few make it a practice to witness their minds at work or stay in the present moment. Besides, staying in the present takes discipline as anyone who tries it knows. There is much to be learned by observing where your mind goes when it wonders and what messages we broadcast. We may even discover how negative we are and that our thoughts can be harmful to others and ourselves. If so, we must go forward with a commitment to see no evil, hear no evil, speak no evil, and especially think no evil. This is imperative if we wish to see improvements.

The world in which we live today is a complicated place. More connected by travel, technology, and communication, the world is full of scientific and humanitarian breakthroughs that have conquered some illnesses and prolonged life. Sadly, it is a more hazardous world. Nuclear proliferation has given many nations the capacity to destroy the world community, and terrorism jeopardizes the security of peace-loving people. Despite material prosperity, many people feel helpless in the large scheme of things. We sometimes find ourselves asking if an individual can do anything about these threatening realities.

We can. First, we can anchor our thoughts in prayer rather than be mired in darkness and without hope. Second, we can own our part in a solution that comes from love, compassion, and forgiveness, and not succumb to what others think or feel when they lead with aggression. Third, we can remember to rein in our ego. Ego is a big factor in how we think and the kind of signals we send out. Since ego thrives on fear, we must try to clear our minds of the negatives that fear creates.

## Sources of Peace and Inspiration

We can seek out sources of peace and inspiration in many ways. One way is through music, which can be soothing and soulful. Play symphonic melodies softly while you are relaxing at home. In his book *The Mozart Effect: Tapping the Power of Music to Heal the Body, Strengthen the Mind, and Unlock the Creative Spirit*, Don Campbell says that "classical music can awaken and stimulate the brain as well as improve listening, and is a stimulus to imagery and visualization."

Another source of peace can be a mantra. A mantra is a phrase or expression that, recited long enough, brings that thought into conscious reality. For instance, you might want to create a phrase and recite it as a source of comfort: "In this day I will seek the highest good for myself and others. God's will be done."

This is one of my personal favorites. This mantra reminds me that God has a design for my life and for everyone, and I remind myself to get out of God's way to let Him guide me where He would have me go. These words remind me to be grateful, to show compassion, and to live in truth, order, and with a sense of purpose in my life.

As an aid to help you manifest good thoughts with powerful results, I have provided a list of words to choose from for your daily mantra.

| | | | |
|---|---|---|---|
| Peace | Joy | Happiness | Truth |
| Love | Beauty | Balance | Harmony |
| Tolerance | Bliss | Compassion | Kindness |
| Understanding | Forgiveness | Inspiration | Soothing |

| Tranquillity | Clarity | Faith | Charity |
| Creativity | Acceptance | Gentle | Soulful |

## Good Thoughts Are Contagious

My friend Alan told me he was at a dinner party when the subject turned to the unfavorable conditions in the stock market. One man suggested that the country was about to slide into a depression, and all the naysayers were talking doom and gloom. Alan decided to insulate himself. He addressed the group, saying as long as he had his health and the love of family and friends, nothing could adversely affect him. Soon everyone within earshot began to talk with hope and optimism. With one voice, one positive, powerful statement, the mood was swayed.

Each of us sends out positive or negative vibrations, often without being conscious that we are doing so. What if we made an effort to be consciously positive, to resonate messages of the highest good for others and ourselves? What if we made a deliberate attempt to keep our thoughts aligned with God's spiritual optimism, to refuse to be stuck in self-centered fear? Our thoughts speak louder than our words. In order to change what we create, we must change our thinking. We must mind our mind.

I like to think of the process of minding one's mind as learning the language of tolerance and compassion. If we become more tolerant and show more compassion, we will speak the new language and carry the powerful messages of change. We thought the world into the place that it's in; now we have to raise the vibration of thought form to help change the world.

CHAPTER 25

# Change You and Change the World

WHEN GOD LOOKS DOWN upon our world, I wonder what He sees. Does He view creation with happy eyes or see a world in need of change? Does He observe a world of justice, harmony, and love or a world lacking in compassion.

If you believe our world needs improvement, I think you are on God's wavelength. The still, small voice that calls many of us to seek fairness and morality, to feed the hungry and clothe the naked, to provide shelter to the homeless, is God's voice urging us to bring into being a more loving world.

How do we bring this kinder and gentler world into being? How do we shift the harsh paradigm of poverty so that we each see ourselves as our brother's keeper? Leo Tolstoy, the nineteenth century Russian novelist who wrote *War and Peace*, observed, "Everybody thinks of changing humanity, but nobody thinks of changing himself." Faced with humanity's problems, we find it's easier to be a critic of the many ills than it is to be a model of what is good. But think about it. When it comes to what we can control, it's much easier to affect our own behavior. Each and every person is a starting point for change.

## The Language of Change

There are three phrases that comprise the language of change.

1. A change of heart is to reverse a previously held emotion or feeling about something or someone.

2. To change one's tune is to alter one's approach or attitude.

3. To change one's mind is to shift a previously held opinion or decision.

Here's an example of how the language works.

It happened the other day, when I was about to get into a verbal confrontation with my friend Scott. I didn't like the way he was behaving about a fairly trivial matter, and I wanted him to change his approach. Just as I was about to unload my anger on him, that voice inside my head suggested I take a time-out and go to the bakery for a cappuccino. While waiting for my coffee, I picked up a flyer and read, "Don't say a word. Think before you speak."

I gasped when I saw the words.

Do I need to tell you that I never confronted Scott with my aggression? Swallowing my destructive anger, I knew that the voice inside my head was God calling and the flyer was God speaking. God was reminding me that if I had a change of heart, I could change my tune. Then by changing my mind, I could affect the outcome of the falling-out I'd had without strife and hostility.

I frequently seek divine insights that help to change my behavior. The key is to stay alert to the signs and wonders, coincidences, and other signals God gives me to show the part I can play in the situation. Through the new language, God speaks to us all the time and we must listen to what He is saying. The process begins when we dedicate ourselves to achieving self-perfection, but in a spirit of humility, remembering to ask God for inspiration.

The God who speaks to me isn't unreasonable. He doesn't tell me to single-handedly clean up the rivers and streams and bring peace on earth to all mankind. Rather, He meets me where I am. Though I may observe the global problems that thwart and even paralyze our world, God knows I am only one person. But I as one person can act locally in my life and sphere of influence to make a great difference. God reminds me not to pollute my back-yard and not to create ill will in my community or with those with whom I interact. It is my sense that He expects me to clean up after myself when I go camping, and He distinctly says, "If you want peace, make peace." Peace on earth begins with how I treat my friends. How can I expect peace in the Middle East if I don't make an effort to make peace with someone I respect and care about?

What sometimes gets in the way of God's messages is our own selfishness and an ego we have to face daily. If I don't start my day on my knees with a prayer, if I don't meditate or daydream into a more centered space, and if I don't write down what's bothering me, my ego takes over. My ego needs but the slightest provocation to engage in the pointless banter of "he said, she said," to puff up his chest and claim to be right about everything. My ego would rather I be right than happy. My ego can get me so angry that I lose my temper. But if I protect myself with the tools of self-reflection and quietude, I can get through the day with peace in my heart, satisfied that I tried my best to find my better nature, even if I failed.

What's your experience with your ego? Does it keep you in con-flict rather than peace? What can you do to clean up the resent-ments and unloving attitudes that you've displayed? How can you become a more peaceful warrior for positive change, to help bring into being the new world of loving kindness that is waiting to be born?

## Healing Our Attitudes

While change is obviously about transformation, we need to know how and where to start. To guide my own behavior, I recently drew up a roster of common problem attitudes that I think harm the world and need healing. Naming these attitudes helped me understand what steps I might take in my personal life to seek a remedy. Opposing each difficult attitude on my list is my remedy. If I can alter my own attitude in these trouble spots in my own life, I can be a part of the solution instead of part of the problem.

*Problem:* Anger
  Anger is a strong feeling of displeasure and antagonism.
*Solution:* Temperance
  Temperance is moderation or restraint in behavior or expression.

*Problem:* Bigotry
  Bigotry is being obstinately or intolerantly devoted to specific opinions and prejudices.
*Solution:* Tolerance
  Tolerance is the capacity or the practice of recognizing and respecting the beliefs or practices of others.

*Problem:* Blaming
  Blaming is finding fault with someone or something or holding that person or thing responsible.
*Solution:* Praising
  Praising is an expression of approval, commendation, or admiration.

*Problem:* Condemnation
  Condemnation is the act of declaring someone or something to be reprehensible, wrong, or evil.

*Solution:* Empathy

Empathy is the capacity for understanding another's feelings or ideas.

*Problem:* Disdain

Disdain is a feeling of contempt or scorn for what is beneath one.

*Solution:* Dignify

Dignify is to raise the status of a person or to confer dignity or honor upon someone.

*Problem:* Disregard

Disregard is treating another as unworthy of consideration and doing so without guilt or remorse.

*Solution:* Consideration

Consideration is heartfelt and thoughtful concern for others.

*Problem:* Dogmatism

Dogmatism is an unwarranted or arrogant viewpoint or system of ideas based on insufficiently examined premises.

*Solution:* Leniency

Leniency is an inclination not to be strict or harsh but to be merciful and generous.

*Problems:* Hatred

Hatred is prejudiced hostility or animosity.

*Solution:* Amicability

Amicability is an exhibition of goodwill or friendliness.

*Problem:* Injustice

Injustice is a violation of the rights of another.

*Solution:* Justice

Justice is the upholding of what is fair and just.

*Problem:* Intolerance

Intolerance is the quality of unwillingness to grant equal free-dom of expression, especially in religious matters.

*Solution:* Tolerance

Tolerance is the quality of willingness to grant equal freedom of expression, especially in religious matters.

*Problem:* Judgmentalism

Judgmentalism is being inclined to pass judgments, especially moral or personal ones.

*Solution:* Nonjudgmentalism

Nonjudgmentalism is being inclined not to make judgments, especially moral or personal ones.

*Problem:* Narrow-mindedness

Narrow-mindedness is lacking tolerance, breadth of view, or sympathy.

*Solution:* Open-mindedness

Open-mindedness is having tolerance, breadth of view, or sym-pathy.

*Problem:* Rage

Rage is violent and uncontrollable anger.

*Solution:* Tranquillity

Tranquillity is the quality of being serene, free from commotion or disturbance.

*Problem:* Revenge

Revenge is an act or instance of retaliating to get even.

*Solution:* Passive Resistance

Passive resistance is resistance by nonviolent methods to a gov-ernment, a person, or an ideology.

*Problem:* Shaming

Shaming is to force a person to action by causing him or her to feel guilty.

*Solution:* Affirming

Affirming is to uphold and support someone's deeds.

*Problem:* Violence

Violence is an exertion of physical force for the purpose of violating, damaging, or abusing another.

*Solution:* Peace

Peace is the state of being undisturbed by strife, turmoil, or disagreement. It is the absence of hostility.

Go over this list of attitudes slowly and carefully. Which ones apply to you? Just for one minute can you see yourself shifting from problem to solution, from a negative attitude to a positive one? Make it your goal to eliminate those negative attitudes that stop you from being part of the powerfully positive world.

For instance, resolve not to have disregard for others. Do not let intolerance and bigotry rob you of joining others to build a better community. Do not let anger and violence send out messages of hate. Create a world of compassion by being compassionate. Create a world of kindness by being kind. Create a world of peace and justice by seeing how alike you are with those whom you consider to be your enemy.

## Seven Steps for Change

Here is a list of seven simple steps for change that have worked for my clients and me. It is my hope that they will work for you too.

1. Pray for the willingness to change. Pray for God's help to change.

Pray for your enemies, locally and globally. Remember that the outcome belongs to God.

2. When you are having difficulties, look within and see what part you played in creating the situation. Whenever possible, meet face-to-face to resolve the disagreement with whomever you are having a dispute.

3. Make a list of your fears. Some fears are intuitive, gut reactions that warn us to be vigilant. But many fears, phobias, and scare tactics are engendered by mass hysteria and need to be seen as phantoms of insecurity, not real concerns.

4. Make a list of your prejudices. Become better acquainted with what causes your bias.

5. Become better educated about people, places, and things that are different. See how ignorance distorts your reason.

6. Seek inspiration from books and music that are uplifting so as to encourage the process of change.

7. Forgive and be forgiven.

## Mary Margaret Learns a Lesson

My friend Mary Margaret was membership chairman for the symphony board where she lived. The president of the guild suggested that Allaya, a newcomer to the community from Pakistan, might serve as cochair with her. Mary Margaret dug in her heels. "I am a Christian and third generation in this town. Nobody knows a thing about that woman." Not only was Mary Margaret close-minded, she apparently had closed her heart as well.

One day in church, her minister preached a sermon on tolerance of others. He said that what causes us to exclude others is fear and ignorance of those whose skin color is different from ours, who pray to a God who is not ours. By the time he ended his talk with "love thy neighbor as thyself," Mary Margaret had opened her mind and heart to change her attitude about Allaya.

"God, please give me a sign of reconciliation," she prayed.

The next day God showed Mary Margaret the way. She saw her two children standing in the schoolyard with Allaya and her children when she came to pick them up. Without hesitation she invited Allaya and her daughters to her house that weekend for a picnic. At the picnic, Allaya asked Mary Margaret to have lunch the next week.

Before the two women got together for lunch, they each investigated the religion and culture of the other through books and tapes and talking to those who were informed about such matters. Mary Margaret learned a lot about what it was like to be a Pakistani and a Muslim, and how hard it was to move to America with conditions in the world being what they were. Allaya read about Episcopalians and New England and through talking with Mary Margaret, learned about what financial hardships she endured growing up in rural Kentucky.

Mary Margaret welcomed Allaya as cochair and gave a tea to introduce her to her women friends.

Mary Margaret initially acted out of fear and ignorance. She was in the grip of global fear of Mideast ethnicity, and she was acting out of ignorance of what she perceived Muslims believed. In a few minutes, over lunch with Allaya, her fear subsided and she learned about what it meant to be a Muslim. They both laughed aloud at how fear and stupidity nearly robbed them of a friendship.

"Mary Margaret, I was just as afraid of you as you were of me. I needed a little education about what Christians believe. We both got a lesson in tolerance. Can you forgive me for my misunderstanding of you?" asked Allaya.

"I already have," said Mary Margaret. "Can you forgive me?"

The women embraced. They had not only settled their differences but found a lot to like in the other.

Today, they are close friends, whose families often travel together. Two of their children are roommates in college.

Change you and change the world.

CHAPTER 26

# The Dawning Age of Miracles

WHAT WOULD THE WORLD be like if each of us were in conscious contact with the divine source? What if we were to get so quiet and clear that the still, small voice inside each of us could make itself heard? What if the signs and wonders, angel murmurs, synchronicities, and coincidences came at us so fast that we would not only hear God's will for our lives but understand how to accomplish it? What if each of us honed our tuning forks to broadcast compassion and tolerance and as it says in the Bible, "provide things honest in the sight of all men"?

If a critical mass of people begin to work with the new language, I believe an extraordinary new era without limits could be ushered in. In this dawning age of miracles, we might witness remarkable changes as many of us got on God's frequency. The channeling of His love and healing energies through us and to others might result in spontaneous healings. Mind-to-mind communication might become the commonplace way of speaking with others as we learned to get on their wavelength. Lying might vanish as our antenna became able to detect and disarm threatening vibrations of deceit or deception as we encountered them.

I admit to being an optimist, but the potential for a new world full of miracles is a vision I hold. Believing in God's unlimited power to work in and through each of us, I see a universe on the cutting edge of greatness following centuries of adversity. Pregnant with the new language, each of us is capable of helping give birth to a world built on an ethic of warmhearted consideration, of dignity and justice. The choice is ours.

To view the new language as a potent catalyst of spiritual change requires recognizing our part in the transition. We have spoken of the need to listen for the sound of divine inspiration, to seek God's guidance and heed it as best we can, and to think pure thoughts. These are the simple steps that can begin a long and rewarding journey.

But in order for the dawning age of miracles to manifest, the sun must set on patterns that have so far deluded us. Our human nature must find the moral high ground to allow our spiritual selves to flourish. Greed must give way to a generosity of spirit, hate must be alchemized into love, and disregard for the plight of others must give way to compassion and understanding. The walls between cultures, nations, races, and social classes must fall—as did the Berlin Wall—allowing a new, improved consciousness to emerge.

How and whether the age of miracles manifests depends upon what we do in our personal lives. If we practice love and tolerance at home and in our neighborhood—at work and at play—our message may radiate out and inspire those on the other side of the globe. If we take responsibility for the messages we are sending out, if we let our heart lead our head, and if we look out for the needs of others as we do for ourselves, I believe the possibilities are infinite. World hunger can end. The billions spent for defense can be allocated to feed our starving brothers and sisters. Homelessness can become a thing of the past. And the fears of the world can shrink.

The delusions of the ego have caused everyday miracles to stop. Part of the prelude to the dawning age of miracles involves putting aside our self-absorption and selfishness, banishing narcissism and fear born of insecurity and the need for excessive control. If we work at doing this, I believe that God will help reunite His children—the prodigals who forgot the language and forgot that God is the loving Father of all of us. The true meaning of this new dawning age of miracles is the recognition that we are divine and are part of one consciousness—we speak the same language without words, a language that springs from the heart to unite us all. We as his children must be ready to live in peace and harmony. And we must desire this age of miracles to dawn.

The opening words of the Declaration of Independence beg consideration as we determine our future relationships at home and abroad. Although this document was our formal separation from the tyranny of England and her king, the sentiment pronounces a commitment to freedom for all.

> When in the course of human events it becomes necessary for one people to dissolve the political bonds which have connected them with another, and to assume among the powers of the earth, the separate and equal station to which the Laws of Nature and of Nature's God entitle them, a decent respect to the opinions of mankind requires that they should declare the causes which impel them to the separation.
>
> We hold these truths to be self-evident, that all men are created equal, that they are endowed by their Creator with certain unalienable Rights, that among these are Life, Liberty and the pursuit of Happiness.

To realize the vision offered by the authors of the Declaration of Independence will take dedication. And it will take prayer. For my own personal inspiration, I never go very long without reading or reciting the Prayer of Peace, attributed to Saint Francis of Assisi but written anonymously during World War I. The Prayer of Peace helps me hold the vision of God's divine plan. Maybe you will also find it helpful as we seek to inherit an age of miracles.

> *Lord, make me an instrument of Thy peace.*
> *Where there is hatred, let me sow love;*
> *Where there is injury, pardon;*
> *Where there is doubt, faith;*
> *Where there is despair, hope;*
> *Where there is darkness, light;*
> *Where there is sadness, joy;*
>
> *O Divine Master, grant that*
> *I may not so much seek*
> *To be consoled, as to console;*
> *Not so much to be understood as to understand;*
> *Not so much to be Loved as to love;*
> *For it is in giving that we receive;*
> *It is in pardoning, that we are pardoned;*
> *It is in dying, that we awaken to eternal life.*

The new millennium of miracles is ours for the asking. To realize its potential, each person must be willing to do his or her part, beginning with a willingness to open up to the power and promise of the new language. Do you feel you are ready to clear away your static? Are you prepared to embrace your ego? Can you find the willingness to change yourself? You are a part of the wondrous creations that are upon us.

CHAPTER 27

# Let the Power Pass

As WE HOPE for the dawning of an age of miracles in our volatile world, each of us has a decision to make. For much too long, our spiritual lives have been governed by a few power brokers who have been all too willing to mediate our relationship with God, telling us what to believe, how and when to pray, and what our holy books say. Through the millennia, these self-anointed middlemen have used the umbrella of organized religion to usurp the right of the people to govern ourselves and to believe what is right for us. Rather than encouraging us to hear what God had to say to us directly, ecclesiastical authorities have suppressed our direct channel to God with harsh pronouncements. As the centuries passed, our adherence to the sanctions of religious bodies not only shaped what we believed but also made us less responsible to ourselves for our actions. Dare I suggest that the anger some feel today toward those of differing religions is transference of their own bottled up rage toward the religious hierarchies that have taken away their power to believe as they so choose?

So then, there is a decision to make. Is it time for you to become your own authority? Is it time for you to be responsible for yourself, to go forth unmediated? And is it time to look to God for direction in your life—to live your life with a universal hope that others may do the same? Only you can decide.

It is my hope that you may have been helped in finding the answers to these questions with the exercises and information found in this book. I hope that you have been helped by what you have learned here about God's unique message system of coincidences, synchronicities, signs and wonders, angel murmurs, omens, epiphanies, and other telepathic ways to communicate. I believe that we all have immediate access to God through the new language, God's mother tongue. I believe you can hear God's guidance and message if you know how to listen.

In our ever-changing universe we are all picking through new ideas, new waves of thought and concepts to see what fits us. If you are at all intrigued by what you have read here, practice the new language in your day-to-day world to solve the mysteries that life presents.

And every day as you stir awake and every night before you shut your eyes to sleep, remember the mantra that can take you to places only God can dream for you: Let the power pass from the few to the many.

# PART V

# Questions and Answers
## About the
## New Language

# CHAPTER 28

# Exploring the New Language

*Is it necessary for me to clear in order to understand the new language?*

No, but it helps. Nearly every adult carries some emotional baggage through life. Our emotions are nothing more than energy that can be light and translucent, like love and joy, or heavy and dense, like fear and anger. Clearing away past resentments and self-destructive emotional patterns actually removes the heavy energy that can hinder our ability to have our own conversation with God, kind of like clearing static on a radio. Our reception of the intuitional messages that come in the new language is diminished when we are angry, upset, worried, or depressed. Our energy fields are too dense at those times and can't receive God's signals that well.

*How long does it take to understand the new language?*

Some of my clients get it right away. For them, it's simply a matter of giving a name to an experience they've been having for a long time. Names really matter, as most of us know. When we read a novel and discover symbolism or go to a movie and witness foreshadowing, we can comprehend the phenomenon more easily because the concept has been identified. It's what C.S. Lewis called the power of naming. The same is true for body language, neurolinguistic programming, and the new language. For a long time, I think, a lot of people were experiencing the mother tongue of God, but they didn't know what to call it. Now that it's been given a name, it will be easier to comprehend.

For those who are slower to hear and use the new language, my advice is to stay with the exercises I have presented in this book, for with practice of prayer, meditation, and journal keeping, you will eventually recognize and speak the new language.

*How long does it take to get fluent in the new language?*

Not long at all, if you are committed. Some of my clients report that once they know the mechanics of the new language, they get into the flow very quickly—usually within a month. They begin to see the interconnectedness of events, people, and signs. In addition, they stop dismissing important guidance as they might have done previously.

*How will I know the difference between my wild and crazy imagination and the new language?*

Great question and one that is often asked. Some of us do have a tendency to read into things, to deceive ourselves, mistaking benign things for divine prompting and guidance. Based on my experience and what my clients tell me, I've concluded that practice is the key that will allow you to delineate between wishful thinking and God's actual hand in your life. Results take time to measure. Besides, when you learn a new language, it's natural to stutter and speak haltingly at first—like baby talk. But there will be real results that will become clearer with time and practice. And I promise you will feel awestruck when you experience them.

*Do you have a simple definition of the new language?*

Yes. Quite simply put, it's God's way of talking to us. The new language is His mother tongue, if you will, the way he's been talking to us since biblical times. Going as far back as Moses and the burning bush, God has been using sign language to get through to us. Now, Moses must have been a very clever fellow because when God showed him a bramble on fire in the middle of the desert, he didn't miss a beat—he marched straight up the mountain to get those Commandments. It's two thousand years later, and the rest of us are still scratching our heads!

*How come?*

After biblical times, organized religions began springing up around the world and there was a power grab. Have you ever noticed how some people like to push other people around? Well, as early religions sprang up, the power became concentrated in a few hands. The people in charge clearly enjoyed telling the rest of the folks what to think and what to do. A great many man-made rules and dogmas were established, and in no time people were down on their knees reciting the "right" prayers at the "right" time of day—as if God were an obsessive-compulsive ego who kept a tight schedule. The God who had made man in His divine image must have had a real chuckle as He watched man remaking Him along human lines.

*Are we still connected to the source while we are on earth?*

Absolutely, and energy is the thread that links everything together. It's the unifying force, the substance out of which all of our emotions and thoughts are made. That's why it is so important to be mindful of what we think and feel, to be constructive with our thoughts and emotions, and not let grievances and ill intentions hang over us. The tiny, energetic pulses radiating out of our hearts and our minds can carry a positive or a negative charge. That charge influences both the force field around us and the larger universe.

*All of this talk about energy places you in Einstein's camp. Are you?*

Yes, life is about energy. When one person is attracted to another, that is energy at work, creating a pull. When someone has charisma, that's energy, too. Laughter is positive energy going out into the universe.

I should stop and interject here that energy is only positive if it is of our highest selves. Energy fueled by a misguided ego can be very dangerous. Hitler, for instance, used great charisma to catastrophic effect by hypnotizing a nation unable to discriminate.

*How do we learn to discriminate?*

That is a very important question with a very simple answer: Ask. Remember that line in the Bible, "Ask and you shall receive"? Well, when you aren't sure if you are with the right people or headed in the right direction, ask for help. Ask often and with an open heart. Throughout each day, check in with God and take note of what you hear, see, or learn. Get sensitive to the new language.

*What do you mean by sensitive?*

More confident and aware. Like any skill, your sensitivity to God's guidance will develop slowly and with practice. That's the journey we have been on in this book—clearing, listening and prac-ticing; we are refining our skills.

*So we are truly created in God's likeness?*

Totally and completely, a true chip off the old energy block. Some of the most important implications of the energy theory are in the areas of health care and medicine. Ever since science began viewing the body as more than flesh and blood, great strides have been made through alternative approaches to medicine, especially the ones that probe deeper into the energy connection. Acupuncture is now used to influence electrical meridians in the body. Magnets affect polarity to treat backaches and bone fractures.

And let's not forget spiritual healing. Through energy points located in hands and through the power of thought, a healer taps into the source of divine energy in order to help the patient recharge his own energy. All of these energy-healing techniques are exciting and can produce extraordinary results.

*There has been much talk in the last few years about people living on in the spirit world after physical death. Does that idea fit in with all this energy talk?*

Very neatly. When the body dies, the soul lives on eternally. That's because the soul is made of energy and energy can be transformed but never destroyed. Once released from its physical container, the soul is free to travel the spirit world, liberated from the rules and regulations of time and space that govern life on earth. But what does a poor soul wear? For such occasions, the etheric body is just the outfit. Our etheric body is an identical copy of our physical body. When people on earth say they have seen someone who has moved on to the spirit world and the person looks more perfect than how they looked on earth, that's because they are appearing in their etheric body. The etheric body is more luminescent and vibrates at a higher frequency of energy than our denser physical body.

*Do you think that people in the spirit world are in any way involved in the new language?*

I do. I believe that our beloved ones sometimes serve as God's messengers. They move things around in our houses and whisper in our ears. I think our thought forms of love pull them to us and they offer what help they can in our day-to-day lives.

*What about angels?*

I'm a believer. God has lots of helpers to get the job done. Angels are messengers from the source.

*In the early part of the century, there was a lot of talk about stream of consciousness. Does God's mother tongue have anything to do with that?*

Yes. You've got it. God's mother tongue, the new language, is part of a divine stream of consciousness. The thoughts in God's head are all around us. We are swimming in them. Once you know this you can move with the tide rather than be taken by the under-tow.

*What about children—can they learn the new language?*

Yes. It is scientifically proven that children pick up foreign languages quicker than adults do. The same is true for learning the new language. Parents often discourage their children's imaginary friends. It is important not to shame children for their vivid imagination or their ability to tune in to their own intuition or a friend's. A major factor in young people being able to hear and speak the new language is being surrounded by adults who reflect an appreciation of it.

PART VI

*Resources*

# About the Sedona Intensive

Incorporated in Sedona, Arizona, more than eighteen years ago, Albert Clayton Gaulden's Sedona Intensive was founded on the belief that God wants all of us to have our own personal tie to Him, to benefit from His direct guidance and love. Gaulden views each person as a channel of communication, and his support team helps individuals clear away the static emotions and difficult upbringings that keep God's voice from reaching each of them.

The Sedona Intensive is not a treatment center but rather a personal-growth program that helps clients face self-destructive compulsions and addictions. The intensive deals with alcoholism and codependency, common problems such as anxiety and depression, as well as divorce and death, by teaching those who go through the process to speak the new language and to free themselves from what troubles them.

The client identifies patterns in his family history that are both emotionally and psychologically damaging—such as secrecy, narcissism, rejection, sexual and physical abuse, and abandonment—through writing and discussing a detailed life inventory, meditating, and journaling. Individuals counsel with a spiritual psychologist, enjoy pampering massages, attend twelve-step meetings, take yoga classes, and receive network chiropractic adjustments. They also breathe through core issues with a transformational breath worker and relax in a Jacuzzi, steam, or sauna after a picturesque hike in the mountains of Sedona. The Sedona Intensive rescues the precious child of God who has been held hostage by his ego. Through the process of clearing—which includes prayer and meditation—the client takes his power back and becomes responsible for his actions.

The books used in the program are *Clearing for the Millennium*, by Albert Clayton Gaulden; *The Invisible Partners: How the Male and Female in Each of Us Affects Our Relationships*, by John A. Sanford; *My Ego, My Higher Power and I: A Transformational Journey from Ego to Higher Self*, by Jerry Hirschfield; *When Things Fall Apart: Heart Advice for Difficult Times*, by Pema Chodron; *Silently Seduced: When Parents Make Their Children Partners: Understanding Covert Incest*, by Kenneth M. Adams, Ph.D; *Why People Don't Heal and How They Can* and *Spiritual Madness: The Necessity of Meeting God in Darkness*, by Caroline Myss; *How to Know God: The Yoga Aphorisms of Patanjali*, by Swami Prabhavananda and Christopher Isherwood; *Answers in the Heart: Daily Meditations*, by the Hazelden Meditation Series; *Words to Live By: Inspirations to Live By*, by Eknath Easwaran and *The Twelve Steps for Everyone . . . Who Really Wants Them*, by Hazelden.

For further information contact:

The Sedona Intensive
P.O. Box 2309
Sedona, Arizona 86339-2309
(928) 282-4723
Web site www.SedonaIntensive.com
Info@SedonaIntensive.com

# Have You Experienced
the New Language?

If you have had an experience with the new language that you'd like to share, please write me:

Albert Clayton Gaulden
The Sedona Intensive
P.O. Box 2309
Sedona, Arizona 86339-2309
stories@SedonaIntensive.com

Watch for your story on my *Sedona Intensive* Web site: www. SedonaIntensive.com.

# Bibliography

Adams, Kenneth M. *Silently Seduced: When Parents Make Their Children Partners: Understanding Covert Incest*. Florida: Heath Communications, Inc., 1991.

Barks, Coleman, and Michael Green. *The Illuminated Prayer: The Five-Times Prayer of the Sufis*. New York: A Ballantine Wellspring Book, 2000.

Bell, Craig S. *Comprehending Coincidence: Synchronicity and Personal Transformation*. West Chester, Pa.: Chrysalis Books, 2000.

Bradshaw, John. *Family Secrets: What You Don't Know Can Hurt You*. New York: Bantam Books, 1995.

Campbell, Don. *The Mozart Effect: Tapping the Power of Music to Heal the Body, Strengthen the Mind, and Unlock the Creative Spirit*. New York: Avon, 1997.

Campbell, Joseph, and Bill Moyers. *The Power of Myth*, ed. Betty Sue Flowers. New York: First Anchor Books, 1991.

Carroll, Lewis. *Alice in Wonderland*. New York: The Platt & Munk Co., 1937.

Coelho, Paulo. *The Alchemist: A Fable About Following Your Dream*, trans. Alan R. Clarke. San Francisco: Harper, 1993.

Coelho, Paulo. *By the River Piedra I Sat Down and Wept,* trans. Alan R. Clarke. San Francisco: Harper Perennial, 1996.

Cousins, Norman. *Anatomy of an Illness as Perceived by the Patient.* Boston: G.K. Hall, 1980.

Davis, Kenneth C. *Don't Know Much About the Bible: Everything You Need to Know About God But Never Learned.* New York: Avon Books, 1998.

Dossey, Larry, M.D. *Healing Words: The Power of Prayer and the Practice of Medicine.* New York: HarperCollins Publishers, 1994.

Dossey, Larry, M.D. *Recovering the Soul: A Scientific and Spiritual Approach.* New York: Bantam Books, 1989.

Fox, Emmet. *Power Through Constructive Thinking.* New York: Harper, 1940.

Fox, Emmet. *The Sermon on the Mount. The Key to Success in Life.* San Francisco: Harper, 1989.

Golsmith, Joel. *The Thunder of Silence,* ed. Lorraine Sinkler. San Francisco: Harper, 1993.

Greeson, Janet. *It's Not What You're Eating, It's What's Eating You.* New York: Pocket Books, 1993.

Guare, John. *Six Degrees of Separation.* New York: Vintage Books, 1990.

Hopcke, Robert H. *A Guided Tour of the Collected Works of C.G. Jung.* Boston and London: Shambhala, 1999.

Hopcke, Robert H. *There Are No Accidents: Synchronicity and the Stories of Our Lives.* New York: Riverhead Books, 1997.

"How to Remember Your Dreams," *Night Light* (1989). San Jose, Calif.: Lucidity Institute.

Jordan, Peter A. "The Mystery of Chance—Jung and Synchronicity," *Strange Magazine.* Rockville, Md.: Strange Magazine Web site, 1997.

Jung, Carl Gustav. *Man and His Symbols*. Westminster, Md.: Double-day, 1969.

Jung, Carl Gustav. *Synchronicity*. Princeton, N.J.: Princeton University Press, 1973.

Jung, Carl Gustav. *The Undiscovered Self*. New York: Back Bay Books, Little Brown and Company, 1957.

Keith, Kent M. and Spencer Johnson. *The Paradoxical Commandments Anyway: Finding Personal Meaning in a Crazy World*. Maui, New York: Riverhead, 2002.

Koestler, Arthur. *The Roots of Coincidence*. New York: Vintage Books, 1973.

M, *The Gospel According to Sri Ramakrishna*, trans. Nikhilananda. New York: Ramakrishna-Vivekananda Center, 1942.

Main, Roderick, ed. *Jung on Synchronicity and the Paranormal*. Princeton, N.J.: Princeton University Press, 1998.

Metzger, Bruce M., and Michael D. Coogan, eds. *Oxford Companion to the Bible*. Oxford: Oxford University Press, 1993.

Myss, Caroline. *Spiritual Madness: The Necessity of Meeting God in Darkness*. Colorado: Sounds True, 1997.

Myss, Caroline. *Why People Don't Heal and How They Can*. Colorado: Sounds True, 1994.

Peck, M. Scott. *People of the Lie: The Hope for Healing Human Evil*. New York: Simon & Schuster, 1983.

Peck, M. Scott. *The Road Less Traveled: A New Psychology of Love, Traditional Values and Spiritual Growth*. New York: Simon & Schuster, 1985.

Pittman, Frank S., M.D. *Man Enough: Fathers, Sons, and the Search for Masculinity*. New York: The Berkley Publishing Group, 1993.

Redfield, James. *The Celestine Prophecy: An Adventure*. New York: Warner Books, 1994.

Sharp, Daryl. *Jungian Psychology Unplugged: My Life as an Elephant.* Toronto, Canada: Inner City Books, 1998.

Shakespeare, William. *Hamlet.* New York: McClure, Phillips, 1901.

Steiner, George. *Language & Silence: Essays on Language, Literature and the Inhuman.* New Haven: Yale University Press, 1998.

Tolle, Eckhart. *The Power of Now: A Guide to Spiritual Enlightenment.* California: New World Library, 1999.

Ulanov, Ann and Barry Ulanov. *Primary Speech: A Psychology of Prayer.* Belleville, Mich.: Westminster John Knox Press, 1988.

Weaver, Warren. *Lady Luck: The Theory of Probability.* New York: Dover, 1982.

# Acknowledgments

I HAVE BEEN FORTUNATE to meet many people who have contributed to my life and my work. I would like to take this opportunity to thank them for their help. This book could not have been written had I not heard and seen the language in the lives of those around me. I will be forever indebted to Joann Davis for helping me discover the New Language, to Leonora Hornblow for helping me refine it, and to Scott Carney for helping me live it.

First I want to acknowledge my mom and dad, and my brothers and sisters, Mary Louise, Bill, Henry, Margie, and Jennie, for teaching me lessons I didn't want to learn.

I want to express my thanks and devotion to my teacher Swami Swahananda for disciplining me to trust what God was saying and for teaching me how to go where He was leading me. A million thanks to Larry Kirshbaum for publishing my first book and continuing to be an angel in my life.

I want to acknowledge Stephen Coslik, who found me through the language of coincidence and supported my work with his employees. And to his wife, Michelle, and his children, Avery and my goddaughter Isabella, for the joy they have brought into my life.

Praise to Steve Kaufman for keeping my computer in high gear while I wrote this book, and to Steve Hansen for designing the excerpt booklet.

I will be eternally grateful to David Arthur Bell for reading the manuscript and giving me his helpful suggestions, and to his wife, Gail, and children Ashley and Andrew for their love and support.

I am appreciative of Joseph De Nucci for understanding the message of *Signs and Wonders* and letting me share it at Miraval, Life in Balance Spa.

I want to thank Unity Church leaders Jane and Jerry Barthalow, Lawrence Palmer, Rebekah Dunlap, and Rev. Dr. Barbara King for spreading the news about the new language.

I want to thank Darrell Harris for being a patient teacher and a loving friend for more than thirty years.

I am grateful to Gay F. Wray, who I met through the language and who has been a wonderful friend for more than seventeen years.

I am obliged to Cindy Nelson and Bill Mullen for teaching me how to love; to Cathy and Paul Friedman, how to laugh; to Gloria and Bob Decker, how to let go; to Kathy G. Mezrano, how to be a kid again; to Carol Marcus, how to comfort; Salle Merrill-Redfield, how to calm down; to Stephanie and John Hogge, how to share; to Diane Ladd and Robert Hunter, how to play; to Joe Braswell, how to feel; to Sagan Lewis, how to forgive; to Kate and John Noonan, how to be a friend; the nuns at the Sarada Convent, how to serve, and to Colin Tapp for showing me the courage to change the things I can.

I want to thank the spiritual lights who paved the way for this book—and none has shone brighter with greater courage than Shirley MacLaine. I want to thank Paulo Coelho, Larry Dossey, Eckhart Tolle, James Redfield and many others, for being torch-bearers of truth and offering touchstones for soul growth.

I am grateful to Ken Davis for his generous help with historical and biblical references. What I didn't remember, he did.

I am indebted to the publisher of Atria Books, Judith Curr, for her vision to publish this book; to Brenda Copeland for kind assistance and quick responses; to the dedicated marketing team Seale Ballenger, Shannon McKenna, and Cathy Gruhn; and most of all, to

Tracy Behar for making the message of this book stronger, clearer, and more audible. Every writer should be so fortunate as to work with such a gifted editor.

I appreciate all of you who sent stories that helped support how God speaks to every one of us.

I am thankful to Rich, Jean, Sabena, Scot and Amy, Garielle, Marc and Jan, Keith and Pamela, Mike, Lois, and other practitioners for the roles they play in making the Sedona Intensive what it is.

To my Saturday-morning support group, my heartfelt thanks for all the love you have given me over the years.

But most of all, to the graduates of the Sedona Intensive, this is your book because you helped me to stay clear enough to write it.

# Index

as omens, 94–95

as premonitions, 93

techniques for recalling and
interpreting, 97–98

## E

Echo effect, 47, 65

Education, role of, 107–8

Edwards, John, 103–4

Ego
defined, 20, 21–22,
140–41
examples of manipulation of,
139–40

Ego deflating
checklist for, 149
examples, 143–44
methods for seeking help,
146–48
negative and positive
qualities, examination of,
144–46
visualization and dialogue
exercise for,
141–43

Einstein, Albert, 8, 111

Energy, 7–9

Enlightenment, 5

Epiphanies, 47–48
dreams as, 93–94

## F

Family
acknowledging your role in,
158–60
negative qualities,
examination of, 152–56
positive qualities,
examination of, 156–58
role of, 151

Father
defects and qualities, examination of, 29–30
story of, 31–32

Faults, listing your, 20–21

Favoritism, family, 152–53

Fear, 106–7

Foreshadowing, 48

Forgiveness
affects of not giving,
171–73
of mother, 26–27
practicing, 179–82
rage letters, writing, 173
role of, 23–27
self, 25–26, 174–79
writing letters of, to others,
174

Fox, Emmet, 23–24, 186–87

Fox, Michael J., 7

Francis of Assisi, Saint,
203–4